The Authoritative Guide to

Grapefruit Seed Extract

ALLAN SACHS, D.C., C.C.N.

THE AUTHORITATIVE GUIDE TO GRAPEFRUIT SEED EXTRACT

LIFERHYTHM

Editor: Peter Greenwood
Cover: Mark Gatter Designs
Layout: Teja Gerken

Library of Congress Cataloging-in-Publication Data
Sachs, Allan.
    The authoritative guide to grapefruit seed extract : a breakthrough in alternative treatment for colds, candida, allergies, herpes, parasites & and various infections / by Allan Sachs.
       p.   cm.
       Includes bibliographic references.
       ISBN 0-940795-17-5
       1. Grapefruit—Seeds—Therapeutic use. 2. Extracts.
I. Title.
RM237.S23 1997
97-44186
615'.32324—dc20
CIP

Copyright © LifeRhythm 1997
       PO Box 806
       Mendocino CA 95460
       Telephone (707) 937-1825 Fax (707) 937-3052
       Printed in the United States of America

*Dedicated to this planet's magnificent
array of microbes:
Sometimes friend, sometimes foe;
Are we not their progeny?
Will they not inherit the earth?*

Author's Advisory

The purpose of this book is to provide information regarding a product commonly referred to as Grapefruit Seed Extract (GSE). Grapefruit Seed Extract is somewhat of a misnomer in as much as GSE is actually a manufactured product synthesized from both the seeds, pulp, and membranous material of grapefruit.

The therapeutic and commercial uses for GSE as herein described have been compiled from the experience of many qualified professionals. However it must be emphasized that the information provided in no way constitutes a recommendation or prescription for the treatment or prevention of ill health. Nor should the information contained within be interpreted as a diagnosis for any condition of ill health. Such functions are the province of qualified healthcare professionals. At present, GSE has not been approved by the United States F.D.A. for the prevention or treatment of any condition of ill health.

It is the express purpose of this book to encourage interest and research into the potential uses of GSE in healthcare and industry. All descriptions of therapeutic or suggested uses is provided for those who are likely to be involved in such research.

Contents

INTRO-
DUCTION

FOR AS LONG AS HUMANS have walked upon the earth, this planet has provided us with an astonishing assortment of natural medicines to help us heal from that which ails us. Earth's pharmacy has included thousands of plant, animal, and mineral substances. Our challenge, once we left the security of our animal instincts, was to discover and promulgate the proper uses of these remedies.

As we entered the twentieth century our pharmacy changed forever. Folk wisdom, and knowledge accumulated over thousands of years was swept away in many areas of the world by the new medicine—pharmaceutical drugs. By then, men of science (women were all but barred from this discipline) had decided that nature's gifts could be copied and even improved upon with synthetic substances—oil and coal tar derivatives created through new techniques in chemistry.

Their conclusions were convincing—pharmaceutical drugs were powerful—in many instances they brought almost instantaneous relief from troubling symptoms. Within a brief thirty years this approach to illness became so dominant that it even expropriated the term "traditional medicine" despite the fact that it was indeed the more radical, experimental, and unproven alternative. Ironically, the term "alternative" is still used for many forms of traditional healing—Chinese and Hindu Ayurvedic systems for example, which have a recorded history of several thousand years.

Most of the early pharmaceuticals were attempts to simulate organic substances, but eventually drugs were created which had no natural counterparts. As medicine strayed further and further from its roots, unmistakable evidence arose showing that these wonder drugs had some very serious drawbacks. Most dramatic were side effects which could in fact be far more serious than the illnesses they were designed to treat. (To this day one of the most common causes of hospitalization is adverse reaction to pharmaceutical drugs, a problem of great concern to scientists of all persuasions.)

In 1969, when I entered the health care field as a research assistant at New York's Downstate Medical

Center, the medical world had all but declared victory over infectious diseases. Students were being taught that with the advancement in our understanding of microbes and an ever increasing array of high tech antibiotics, disease causing germs would eventually go the way of the dinosaur. Although some infectious diseases have now been quelled, today there are many germ induced conditions which only twenty-five years ago did not exist or were not yet identified.

When I began working with patients as a clinician in 1977, little attention was paid by practitioners or the public to Chronic Fatigue Syndrome, Cytomeglovirus, AIDS, Epstein Barr Virus Syndrome, Lyme's disease, genital herpes and genital warts. And although Dr. Orion Truss had elaborately and accurately described the disastrous effects of the yeast Candida albicans on many of his patients, few took him seriously. The last twenty years has seen an exponential increase in the number of people suffering from parasitic diseases, a result of increased international travel and a burgeoning immigrant populace in the Americas. In 1977 Giardia lamblia, Entamoeba histolytica, Blastocystis hominis, and Cryptosporidium were of no great concern to Americans; now half of our domestic water supplies are suspected of carrying unacceptable levels of disease causing bacteria and protozoa.

To that list we can add flesh eating bacteria (a mutant form of *Staphlococcus aureus)*, rampant cases of bacterial food poisoning, and a resurgence of some diseases, such as tuberculosis, previously thought to be under control.

With each of these new conditions a host of new pharmaceutical antibiotics sprang up ready to wage war against them. As a physician trained in holistic healthcare, I viewed the medical world's total dependence upon these pharmaceutical solutions with a good deal of suspicion. After all, it had been demonstrated that the promiscuous use of pharmaceutical antibiotics played a significant role in the development of some of the aforementioned diseases.

My search for safe, botanically derived products which could be used, when appropriate, in place of the more toxic pharmaceutical antibiotics, eventually led me, in 1991, to Grapefruit Seed Extract (GSE), a substance derived from the seeds, membranes, and pulp of the grapefruit. It was reputed to be highly effective as a purifier, preservative, and antiseptic and to have extraordinary potential for inhibiting fungi, viruses, and bacteria. My experience and research since then has corroborated those claims. I have used GSE extensively in my practice and in many ways it has changed my approach to health care both personally and professionally. And I am certainly not alone in my appreciation of its properties—a rapidly increasing number of physicians throughout the world now routinely recommend GSE and they report excellent clinical results.

Despite the profound influence that GSE has had upon the holistic approach to disease causing microbes, most of our formal knowledge about it is derived from isolated scientific studies. This book presents my personal and professional experience with GSE and consolidates much important research of interest to the holistic health practitioner and the consumer.

It is my hope that this book will inspire further reseach on this versatile substance as well as assist in the paradigm shift many of us fervently seek. In that regard, Grapefruit Seed Extract has the potential for showing us how nature and science can work in harmony for a healthier world.

Chapter

1

A B O U T
S E E D S

PICK A FRUIT, any fruit—an apple for instance. Bury it in fertile soil. Now the miracle of nature's recycling plan begins. Within seconds, millions of microscopic fungi, bacteria, and protozoa (one-celled animals) can be found on the outer surface. Whether there simply by chance contact, or by *chemotaxis* (the movement of a living organism by chemical attraction or repulsion), the microbes employ all of their chemical forces to penetrate the peel of the apple. With the help of the warm earth and its available nutrients, the microbes multiply into the billions in a matter of hours as the apple itself contributes to the nutrient pool.

Once the peel is breeched the flesh goes quickly. Within a few days the apple is almost unrecognizable.

But then the miniscule invaders hit a snag; little black seeds, holding all the genetic information required for reproduction, put up a fierce resistance.

Not only do these seed have a tough shell, but they have another form of protection: powerful chemicals on the order of cyanide and strychnine repel the invaders time and time again. But the microbes are relentless, sacrificing millions of their kind in the struggle. Eventually the seeds soften, the "bug repellents" expire and the microbes have their final feast. Except, that is, for a few seeds tough enough to resist: these survivors will sprout!

Now had you buried a grapefruit (or any other citrus fruit), the story would have been quite different. Right from the beginning the microbes would have met a mighty resistance. The peel of the grapefruit is not only thick, but it contains powerful chemical deterrents such as limonene, linalol, and citral aldehyde. The microbes must wait: time is on their side. But how much time?

Weeks go by. Finally, due to dehydration, the peel begins to crack. The microbes press on, only to be met by a powerful array of scorching acids and biochemicals issued from the pulp and membranous material. Whereas the apple succumbed in couple of weeks, the grapefruit hangs on for months. The number of tiny lives lost in the assault is staggering. But eventually the invading microbes reach the seeds and the end is near. Or is it?

The seeds are quite soft, seemingly vulnerable. But nature puts a high priority on protecting precious genetic material. In this case the polyphenolic compounds that abound in the seed serve as dedicated palace guards. The scene is now littered with bacteria, fungi, and protozoa all dying for the last bit of fruit. The outstanding ability of citrus fruit to withstand the decaying process is well known to organic gardeners; citrus is generally considered unsuitable for composting unless the gardener is willing to wait almost two years for it to properly decay.

Why is all this of such interest to a health practitioner like myself? Because of one curious fact: while the organic germ inhibiting chemicals derived from most seeds can be quite toxic to humans and animals, the polyphenolic compounds contained in the grapefruit seed and membrane can be converted into a form that retains its natural antimicrobial properties and is virtually non-toxic to human life. In the next chapter we will take a closer look at this form and its ability to combat various bacteria, fungi, parasites, and viruses.

2

A B O U T

GRAPEFRUIT

S E E D

EXTRACT

GRAPEFRUIT SEED EXTRACT (GSE) is a broad spectrum, non-toxic, antimicrobial product derived from the seeds, pulp and white membranes of grapefruit*. In hundreds of laboratory tests, GSE has demonstrated its ability to kill or inhibit the growth of a wide array of potentially harmful bacteria, fungi, viruses and protozoan parasites (Table 2, end of chapter, presents a selected list of microbes tested). These studies have been conducted *en vitro* (in test tubes and petri dishes). Although the more costly *en vivo* studies (on living subjects) have so far been limited to acute toxcity studies, reports from health care practitioners worldwide indicate that GSE has important clinical applications.

---

*GSE is not to be confused with products containing bulking agents made from the pulp fiber of grapefruit or various citrus extracts used in cleansers, deodorizers, etc.

In addition to its broad-spectrum antimicrobial properties, GSE is effective at very low levels of concentration. (see Table 2). Studies comparing GSE with chlorine bleach, isopropyl alcohol, and colloidal silver (see Ch. 9) have consistently found GSE to be superior as an antimicrobial.

What is Grapefruit Seed Extract?

The extract itself is derived by converting large amounts of grapefruit seeds, membranes and pulp into a highly acidic liquid.   This starting material is an excellent source of polyphenolic compounds such as quercitin, hesperidin, neohesperidin, campherol glycoside, naringin, apigenin, rutinoside, poncirin, etc. The polyphenols themselves are unstable but are chemically converted into more stable substances that belong to a diverse class of compounds called *quaternary ammonium products* or 'quats'.

Some quaternary compounds, *benzethonium chloride* and *benzalkonium chloride* for example, are used industrially as antimicrobials but are toxic to animal life. The B vitamin choline is also a quat (as is vitamin B1) but it is non-toxic and essential for maintaining healthy neurological function and fat metabolism. The chemical structure of the quaternary ammonium compounds produced from GSE has not yet been fully elaborated but it appears that the newly formed quaternaries feature the best of both worlds—they are highly antimicrobial, but when used appropriately appear to be nontoxic.

The resulting liquid product is extremely acidic and bitter (a quality viewed by practitioners of Chinese and Ayurvedic medicine as a part of the therapeutic function) therefore pure vegetable glycerine (forty to fifty percent) is added to reduce the acidity and bitterness. The final result—Grapefruit Seed Extract—is a processed product derived from natural sources.

Table 1 presents the properties of GSE. The proportions and figures given here may vary slightly because no two manufacturers of GSE make an identical product.

TABLE 1*

Grapefruit Extractive	*60%*
Glycerine	*40%*
Chemical description	*diphenol hydroxy-benzene complex*
Form of liquid	*viscous*
Color (Gardner)	*2, Lemon yellow*
Odor	*mild citrus*
Specific gravity (dc 25° C)	*1.110*
Density (lbs/gal.)	*9.68*
*pH** (25°)*	*2.0–3.0*
*Flashpoint****	*292 degrees F*
Molecular weight	*565*
*Viscosity***** (Centistoke)*	*144.91*
Solubility	*water, alcohol, and organic solvents*

This 60/40 mix is called 'Standardized Extract of Grapefruit'. It is extremely acidic and should be used only under the supervision of a qualified practitioner. To moderate its highly caustic quality, some manufacturers dilute the 'Standardized' mix with an equal amount

---

* Provided by Biochem Research, Lakeport, California

** pH: degree of acidity/alkalinity on a scale of 0-14 with 7 representing a neutral state. A pH lower than 7 represents an acidic compound; above 7 represents an alkaline state. A pH of 2.0–3.0 for GSE is comparable to the level of acidity of hydrochloric acid found in the human stomach.

*** Flashpoint: the temperature at which a liquid releases enough vapor to form an ignitable mixture with the air above its surface.

**** Viscosity index: a scale indicating a liquid's resistance to flow; the higher the rating the slower the flow. The viscosity presented above is close to that of pure glycerine.

of vegetable glycerine thus creating a product which contains 50% 'Standardized Extract' and 50% vegetable glycerine. This concentration is still sufficiently potent but safer to use; it is the mix called for in all treatment suggestions given in this book. GSE is available in other concentrations, therefore if the consumer is using one other than the fifty/fifty mix, it will be necessary to convert the recommended doses (see the Conversion Table on page 124).

GSE is also made in powder form suitable for encapsulation. It is nearly devoid of any unpleasant bitter taste and because it is considerably less acidic than the liquid concentrate it is preferred for certain applications. The powder (made by spraying silicon dioxide with a fine mist of GSE liquid) is a fine white substance with little odor or taste. It contains approximately:*

Total Grapefruit Extractive   50%
Vegetable Glycerine   20%
Silicon dioxide   30%

The ability of a substance to prevent the growth of a particular germ strain can be assessed, quantified and stated as a of its Minimum Inhibitory Concentration (MIC), the most commonly used laboratory measure of an antimicrobial's effectiveness. The MIC is the *least amount of a substance required to prevent the growth of a microbe under laboratory conditions.*

---

* Information supplied by Biochem Research, Lakeport, California

The MIC is usually stated in parts per million (ppm). A low number, such as 3 ppm, indicates that a given antimicrobial is very effective at inhibiting the growth of the microbe tested. A MIC of 2000 would indicate the need for one part of antimicrobial in 500 parts solution; a MIC of 20,000 parts per million (one part in fifty) indicates far less effectiveness, but it may still be useful under certain circumstances where it would be feasible to use a high concentration.

The MIC does not indicate the ability of a substance to kill a microbe. That rating can be expected to be somewhat higher. However, for many clinical applications the ability to inhibit the growth of a microbe is tantamount to killing it.

Table 2 is a list of those microbes with the significant clinical implications. Tests were performed using the aforementioned Standardized Extract of Grapefruit.* The figures given should be viewed with an allowance for GSE make-up and other testing variables.

TABLE 2**

Gram Negative Bacteria	Origin	Strain #	Mic
Brucella abortus	NCTC	8226	2
Escherichia (E) coli	NCTC	86	2
Haemophilus influenzae	A		660
Klebsiella pneumoniae	ATTC	4352	6
Legionella pneumoniae	isolate		200

* The results provided do not necessarily indicate effectiveness in a clinical setting. En vivo testing with live subjects would be required in order to fully evaluate GSE's clinical usefulness.
** Table provided by Biochem Research, Lakeport, California.

Gram Negative Bacteria (Continued)	Origin	Strain #	Mic
Neisseria catarrhalis	NCTC	3622	660
Pasteurella septica	NCTC	948	2
Proteus vulgaris	NCTC	8313	2
Pseudomonas aeruginosa	NCTC	1999	2000
Salmonella enteritidis	A		6
Salmonella typhi	NCTC	8384	6
Shigella dysenteriae	NCTC	2249	2
Vibrio cholerae	A		200
Gram Positive Bacteria			
Clostridium botulinum	NCTC	3805	60
Clostridium tetani	NCTC	9571	60
Corynebacterium- diptheriae	AtCC	6917	60
Diplococcus pneumoniae	NCTC	7465	60
Listeria monocytogenes	ATCC	15313	20
Mycobacterium- tuberculosis	A		2000
Staphlococcus aureus	NCTC	4163	2
Streptococcus pyogenes	NCTC	8322	60
Streptococcus viridans			20
Fungi and Yeast			
Candida albicans	ATCC	10259	60
Monilla albicans			10
Trichophytum- mentagrophytes	ATCC	9533	20
Trichophytum rubrum	A		200

GSE has also been tested against the following micro-organisms and shown to be effective (under laboratory conditions) at relatively low concentrations; the MIC has not yet been determined.

Campylobacter jejuni
Chlamydia trachomatis
Entamoeba histolytica
Giardia lamblia
Herpes simplex virus type 1
Helicobacter pylori
Influenza A2 virus

HOW DOES
GRAPEFRUIT SEED EXTRACT WORK?

The precise mechanism by which a therapeutic substance exercises its influence is often the last aspect to be understood. The most often quoted example of this is aspirin. Since its development in 1899, aspirin's effects have been experienced by billions of people—the scientific studies on aspirin alone would fill many volumes. Nevertheless, exactly how aspirin works its magic to lower fever and reduce inflammation and pain is only now coming to light. It is therefore not surprising that we are far better able to describe the beneficial effects of GSE than precisely how those benefits are obtained.

Recently however, the remarkable efficacy of GSE has spurred world-wide interest: from Seoul, Korea, Dr. Sung-Hwan of Abcom Chemie Co., LTD states:

> *Considering all the electron micrographs, we believe that the microbial uptake of GSE alters the cell membrane (the envelope surrounding living cells—author) by inhibiting enzymatic activities....You can see the loss of the cytoplasmic membrane.*

These findings appear to corroborate the work of Dr. Roger Wyatt, associate professor at the University of Georgia, who has performed extensive research on GSE as an organic disinfectant. While observing the deactivation of the cytoplasmic membranes of bacteria, Dr. Wyatt was also impressed by GSE's lack of toxicity:

> *The lack of significant toxicological properties of GSE is also impressive when one views the efficacy data...extremely small concentrations of the product can be used with marked beneficial results.*

Of course the next area of inquiry would be the mechanism by which GSE affects the cell membranes of such a diverse group of microbes with virtually no toxicity to animal life. Furthermore, since viruses have no cell membrane of their own, the antiviral properties of GSE remain a mystery. Although the mechanism(s) of action of GSE must indeed be intriguing to microbiologists, there is little money available for the research of non-patentable remedies. Unraveling the intricacies of GSE's functioning will provide much useful knowledge regarding the basic biology of microbes; let us hope that the compelling nature of these questions accelerates the search for these answers.

THE DISCOVERY OF
GRAPEFRUIT SEED EXTRACT

Like so many profound discoveries, the story of GSE began with a simple question. Jacob Harich was eating a grapefruit for breakfast one morning in France and savoring its taste. World War II had just ended and since fresh fruit was a rare treat in Europe at that time, Jacob savored it all the more—until, that is, he bit into a seed! The extremely bitter taste of the seed, interrupted his enjoyment but also prompted a question: "What makes the grapefruit seed so bitter?" For many, such a question might merely have been rhetorical, but for Jacob, a budding scientist, it inspired one of the more compelling inquiries of modern science. This search spanning several decades, is only now bearing fruit and bearing it in many surprising ways.

Jacob Harich was born in Yugoslavia in 1919 and educated in Germany. World War II interrupted his studies in nuclear physics. After witnessing the horrors of war as a fighter pilot, young Harich was inspired to devote the rest of his life to improving the human condition. To this end he augmented his studies with a full university education in medicine, specializing in gynecology and immunology. Upon emigrating to the United States in 1957, Dr. Harich furthered his education at Long Island University (New York). But it wasn't until 1963, after moving to Florida, the heart of grapefruit country, that he received the necessary support to carry out his research.

Dr. Steven Otwell and Dr. Wayne Marshall, both of the University of Florida at Gainesville, are leading researchers on the effects of microbes on food. Although initially skeptical about Dr. Harich's claim of a remarkable organic antimicrobial derived from grapefruit, they were quickly won over by the astonishing capacity of GSE to protect fruit, vegetables, poultry, and fish from the assault of bacteria, fungi, and parasites. The reputation of these two doctors and the renown of Gainesville's food science laboratory prompted other prestigious institutions to give serious consideration to Dr. Harich's claims.

Dr. Harich's work with GSE received a great boost in 1990 as holistic health practioners in the United States began to understand the implications of GSE's antimicrobial capabilities. Finally, after more than a quarter of a century of investigation, Dr. Harich's life work had found the ear of the scientific world.

In 1995 Dr. Harich was invited to Europe as a guest of honor of the Pasteur Institute of France, Europe's leading AIDS research center. For several years the Institute has been researching the potential of GSE as a prophylaxis against the HIV virus as well as against some of the secondary infections associated with AIDS. He was also honored by farmers in Europe who now use a powdered form of GSE in fish and poultry feed to fight two potentially lethal bacteria: Salmonella and E. Coli.

Dr. Harich made himself available to researchers from around the world; in 1995 I had the pleasure of interviewing him in his hometown of Castlebury, Florida. His enthusiasm for research and discovery had not waned despite his years and his upcoming agenda included many new research projects involving GSE. I was saddened to learn of Dr. Harich's passing in May of 1996. Surely the recognition he ultimately received for his pioneering work must have been greatly satisfying to a man who devoted half his life to the development of a revolutionary approach to the control of dangerous germs

Chapter

3

THE
ADVANTAGES
OF
GRAPEFRUIT
SEED
EXTRACT

I N JULY OF 1990, a year before I had learned of GSE, I developed a set of criteria by which to judge the desirability of antimicrobials. I did this at the request of a nutritional supplement manufacturer who considered me qualified because of my previous work as a medical researcher and my experience as a clinical practitioner. To achieve a higher level of objectivity, I polled several of my colleagues and arrived at ten important attributes of an ideal antimicrobial.

Since 1991, my experience as a practitioner, and the experience of the many physicans and hundreds of patients with whom I have spoken, has convinced me that GSE is, according to these criteria, a superior antimicrobial.

Ten Criteria for Judging an Antimicrobial
applied to
Grapefruit Seed Extract

1. Broad Spectrum

Since we rarely can be certain of the exact germ, or mix of germs, is the target of our control effort, it is important that an antimicrobial work against a wide range or *broad spectrum* of microbes. GSE's extraordinary ability to perform against harmful bacteria, fungi, viruses and protozoa is attested to in Table 2 (Ch. 2) which lists some of the microbes known to be inhibited by GSE.

2. Powerful and Effective

Laboratory studies have repeatedly shown that GSE is effective against dangerous germs even when it is greatly diluted; typically, only two hundred to two thousand parts per million are required. (See Table 2, Ch. 2)

3. Non-toxic

Studies have shown GSE to be safe and non-toxic even at dosages many times the recommended amount. An acute toxicology study performed by the Northview Pacific Laboratory (July, 1995) reported that GSE appears safe at levels "exceeding 5000 mg. per kg. of body weight." Hence a person weighing sixty kilograms (132 lbs.) would theoretically be safe with a dose of 300,000 mgs. per day, a preposterously huge dose since typical consumption is less than 1,000 mgs. per day.

4. Minimal Negative Impact on Beneficial Bacteria

While massive doses of GSE are likely to compromise beneficial flora such as Lactobacillus and Bifidobacterium residing in the digestive and urogenital tracts, typically recommended doses of GSE do not appear to have this effect. GSE may actually assist the growth of the beneficial bacteria by inhibiting pathogenic microbes which compete with the beneficial flora.

5. Well Researched

More than eighty scientific laboratories have performed hundreds of studies on the effectiveness of GSE (see list of labs at end of chapter). These studies regularly confirm the broad spectrum activity of GSE when it is taken in proper dosages. However, clearly more research regarding its clinical uses and safety needs to be performed.

6. Derived from Natural Sources

GSE is derived from natural plant material, a factor seen by most holistic practitioners as an advantage over complex production techniques used to derive antibiotics from petroleum and coal tar. It is true however, that some pharmaceutical antibiotics are derived from nature—eg. penicillin from bread mold.

7. Hypo-allergenic

For many years the leading cause of death from prescription drugs was *anaphylactic shock* (a severe reaction leading to circulatory failure) brought on by penicillin and penicillin-type antibiotics. Allergic reactions to other prescription antibiotics, while usually less severe, are so common that many patients have to moderate or switch to a different family of antibiotics. GSE, even if taken on a regular basis, rarely produces a significant allergic reaction. However, since GSE is quite acidic, it may irritate an already distressed stomach or intestinal lining.

8. Biodegradable

Just as we need to respect the natural order of our own internal environment, so do we need to be responsible to the earth's ecosystem. This is especially true when antibiotics are used for commercial purposes. Since the world of commerce is finding new and ingenious ways to employ GSE, it is particularly important that this new approach not further upset the delicate balance of nature we too often take for granted.

It is therefore comforting to know that on August 31, 1994, Bio Research Laboratories of Redmond, Washington, confirmed the biodegradability of GSE. According to this highly regarded facility, the extract was tested under conditions utilizing "standard test methods for determining the anaerobic biodegradation potential of organic materials." They concluded that due to its organic structure, "GSE appears to pose no threat to the environment."

9. Compatible with other Natural Remedies

Chinese herbal medicine, a tradition spanning 5,000 years, has shown that herbal combinations are often more beneficial than single herb remedies. The advantages of the synergistic effects of GSE are attested to by the fact that over seventy-five different herbal combination formulas containing GSE are now available. In addition, GSE's antimicrobial power makes it an excellent preservative thus enabling the herbs it accompanies to retain their potency.

10. Affordable

A typical GSE treatment costs between fifty and seventy-five cents per day—extremely economical compared with prescription antibiotics. GSE is derived from an inexpensive source—grapefruit seeds and pulp which, until recently, were discarded. Furthermore, because it is so efficient, only a small amount is generally required.

LABORATORIES*

ABC Research, Gainesville, Florida
Abcom Chemie Co., Seoul Korea,
Alpha Chemical and Biomedical Laboratories, Petaluma, California
AquaLandis Inc., Canada
Analytical Chemical Services Inc., Columbia, Maryland
Association of Consulting Chemists and Chemical Engineers
Bioassay Systems Corp., Woburn, Massachusetts
Bio-Research Laboratories, Redmond, Washington
Brigham Young University, Provo, Utah

*A partial list of labs that have tested GSE since 1974.

British Columbia Research Corp., Vancouver, B.C., Canada
Coopemontecillos Division Pesca, San Jose, Costa Rica
Daiwa Kasei Chemical, Tokyo, Japan
Department of Health and Human Services, FDA, Washington, D.C.
Department of Food Technology, Gycongsang National University, Chinju, Korea
East Chilliwack Agricultural Co-op, Chilliwack, B.C., Canada
Great Smokies Labs., Asheville, North Carolina
Florida Department of Agriculture, Tallahassee, Florida
Hazelton Labs., Madison, Wisconsin
Hilltop Research Inc., Miamiville, Ohio
ImuTech Inc., Huntington Valley, Pennsylvania
Indonesian Government at the National Center for Fisheries, Jakarta
Institut Pasteur, Paris, France
Journal of Food Sciences
Journal of the Korean Agricultural Chemical Society
Journal of Orthomolecular Medicine
Lancaster Laboratories, Lancaster, Pennsylvania
Northview Pacific Labs, Berkeley, California
Silicon Valley Chemlab Inc., Santa Clara, California
Thornton Laboratories Inc., Tampa, Florida
U.S. Dept of Agriculture, Hyattsville, Florida
United States Testing Co., Hoboken, New Jersey
Universidad Autonoma de Nuevo Leon, San Nicolas de los Garza, Mexico
Universidad National Mayor de San Marcos, Lima, Peru
University of California, Davis, California
University of Florida, Food Services Dept., Gainesville, Florida
University of Nebraska
University of Southern Florida, Dept. of Biology, Tampa, Florida
Valley Microbiology Services, Palo Alto, California
Weston-Gulf Coast Laboratories, University Park, Illinois.

Chapter

4

THE PROBLEMS WITH PHARMA- CEUTICAL ANTIBIOTICS

SINCE THE DISCOVERY of penicillin in 1929, scores of pharmaceutical antibiotics have been brought to market. Some of them have been available for years, but many are no longer prescribed because they either created more problems than they solved, were relatively ineffective, or because the microorganisms they were designed to inhibit developed a resistance to them.

As reports from independent researchers come to light, it becomes more apparent that there may be serious drawbacks to the use of almost every prescription antibiotic studied. There is no question that pharmaceutical antibiotics have saved many lives (they are certainly necessary under many circumstances); rather it is the promiscuous use of these drugs that must be questioned.

ABUSE OF ANTIBIOTICS

In the United States, it has been estimated that a typical three-year old child has had approximately ten courses of antibiotics (most often for ear infections) consisting of two doses per day for ten days making a total of 200 doses. To this astounding figure add another two courses per year (a conservative figure) for the next eight or nine years—an additional 320 doses. Thereafter, with dental procedures, colds, flus, surgeries, etc. many people will receive at least one course of antibiotics per year, again averaging two doses for ten days. A person consuming antibiotics at that rate will have consumed over *1,000 doses* by the age of fifty! Let's now look at some adverse effects that result from the abuse of antibiotics.

TOXICITY

Excessive exposure to metabolic poisons (toxins), so prevalent today due to pollutants in our food, air, and water, contributes significantly to immune suppression and thereby leaves the body vulnerable to infection as well as chronic degenerative processes. By using toxic chemical antibiotics to fight germ induced diseases we only perpetuate a vicious cycle. Antibiotics such as Ketoconazole, Diflucan, and Nizarel are potentially so toxic that patients using them must be continuously monitored for liver damage. Recent studies have shown that if certain anti-histamines are taken with the afore-mentioned antibiotics grave consequences may ensue.

Streptomycin, once routinely prescribed, is now used in only the most dire of situations because of its toxicity. Penicillin was for many years the leading cause of pharmaceutical drug-related deaths; tetracycline, (a successor of penicillin) has been known to cause permanent yellow staining in the teeth of young children. Furthermore, questions remain about the relationship of tetracycline to certain forms of cancer.

Ironically, Erythromycin, commonly prescribed for ear infections in children, has been implicated as the cause of hearing loss in some of those treated. Even Nystatin, the antifungal drug generally prescribed for Candida albicans infection, and considered one of the safest of antibiotics, is often extremely upsetting to the digestive tract; many patients cannot tolerate this anti-biotic.

IMMUNE SUPPRESSION

Medical researchers generally agree that most prescription antibiotics suppress the immune system (practicing physicians often ignore this fact of basic research). The toxic effect of the drugs often weakens some of the organs (thymus, spleen, liver, adrenals) most needed to fend off potentially harmful microbes. Furthermore the die-off of the microbe can be so rapid that the body is unable to program against the germ thus creating a greater likelihood of relapse.

This is most apparent in the treatment of sore throat caused by Beta hemolytic streptococcus. Antibiotics are used by conventional physicians as an early intervention for strep throat to prevent the immune system from producing antibodies which can, in rare instances (less than one in two hundred), cause heart and kidney damage. However, interference with the natural immune response may leave the patient vulnerable to repeated strep infections. Parents who see their children coming down with one sore throat after another with the attendant swelling of the tonsils, can attest to this phenomenon.

DESTRUCTION OF BENEFICIAL BACTERIA

Just as pharmaceutical antibiotics kill harmful bacteria, so do they all too often destroy certain species of bacteria essential to our health. Lactobacillus acidophilus and Bifidobacterium bifidus (found in the digestive and urogenital tracts) are two of perhaps twenty or more such beneficial microbes. They are essential to proper digestion, assimilation, detoxification, vitamin production, hormone processing, cholesterol control, and cancer prevention.

These probiotic cultures also produce natural antibiotics and powerful antifungal enzymes; in the digestive tract they are our first line of defense against harmful bacteria, yeast, and viruses. When pharmaceutical antibiotics weaken or destroy these symbiotic bacteria, persistent yeast infections and bacterial imbalance are likely to follow. For this reason holistic healthcare practitioners look upon the long term use of tetracyline for treating acne in adolescents as one of the great follies of modern medicine. Since most cases of acne can be treated successfully with dietary modification, vitamin therapy, and botanically derived antimicrobials (including GSE), it is difficult to justify destroying intestinal flora in an attempt to treat acne. I have seen scores of Candida sufferers whose problems stemmed from years of tetracyline abuse.

CREATION OF MUTANT MICROBES

It is universally acknowledged that pharmaceutical antibiotics are a primary factor in creating mutant, and often more dangerous, microbes. One mechanism for this is natural selection—survival of the fittest. In any large population of microorganisms there is usually enough genetic variation to allow a small percentage to survive even the most powerful drug. If the conditions are right, these hardy survivors have the potential to develop a whole new super strain—one with a significantly higher resistance to that drug. While this resistance was once thought to be specific to a single drug or family of drugs (e.g., antibiotics containing sulphur), it now appears that certain strains are capable of using this "learning experience" to become immune to other antibiotics. The "doomsday germ" of science fiction movies might be closer than we would like to imagine.

Scientists have now identified several potentially deadly strains of bacteria which are all but impervious to every known antibiotic. For instance, a strain of Staphlococcus aureus that is resistant to Vancomycin (one of the most powerful antibiotics ever developed) has received great notoriety as a "flesh-eating bacteria" responsible for several deaths in the U.S. and Europe. This bacteria is so aggressive that death may ensue in a matter of days despite the best efforts of medicine.

Drug resistant germs are a fact of life in the medical practitioner's office. Gonorrhea, a sexually transmitted disease, is a classic example. Once easily controlled, the offending bacteria (Gonococcus neiseria) is now unaffected even by massive doses of penicillin. Newer pharmaceutical antibiotics are beginning to face the same problem with this insidious disease. And we are beginning to see drug resistant cases of tuberculosis, a disease thought to have been under control but now reappearing, particularly in large cities where the risk is increased by overcrowded conditions.

Pharmaceutical antibiotics also appear to promote mutant strains through a process more direct than natural selection. It now appears that some drugs are capable of directly promoting genetic mutations both in the chromosomes of patients and in the genetic programming of the microbe. Most of the genetic material of a microbe resides within the nucleus. However plasmids (cell organs outside of the nucleus), also contain genetic information (DNA). Researchers have discovered a complex system by which microbes can exchange genetic material through these plasmids—even from one species to another. It is believed that the resistance of certain strains of E. coli to Vancomycin has already been transferred to Staphloccocus aureus thereby producing the aforementioned "flesh eating bacteria."

In September of 1995, the American Medical Association finally began to put its weight against the overuse of antibiotic drugs. The A.M.A. declared the promiscuous use of antibiotics a serious health problem not only to those who consumed them, but also a threat to the health of everyone because they may produce dangerous mutant strains of microbes. To reduce this risk, the A.M.A. has proposed to launch programs that would teach doctors how to be more discriminating in their use of antibiotics.

As we continue our research into the world of botanical substances, our reliance on synthetic drugs might decrease. Garlic, for example, has been used for thousands of years to control a broad range of dangerous microbes with virtually no side-effects. And now we have a new ally from the plant kingdom: Grapefruit Seed Extract.

5

GRAPEFRUIT SEED EXTRACT IN MY PRACTICE

AS A NATURAL HEALTH CARE practitioner and medical researcher, I have had a long standing interest in alternatives to pharmaceutical antibiotics. In 1991 this interest prompted me to attend a conference on holistic approaches to digestive disorders. The event was chaired by Dr. Leo Galland, M.D. of New York City. Dr. Galland's impeccable medical credentials and his pioneering work on the environmental causes of illness have made him a leading spokesman in holistic health care. I had read Dr. Galland's account of Grapefruit Seed Extract, a new product he used to control a wide range of harmful microbes; it was my introduction to GSE. Here are some of Dr. Galland's remarks regarding his experience with GSE:

It would be hard for me to overestimate the value of GSE in my medical practice. This broad spectrum, antimicrobial product has no inherent toxicity except for a concentration-dependent local irritant effect.... For years I have used GSE in the treatment of intestinal parasitism and chronic candidiasis with excellent results. It appears as effective as Nystatin (the most commonly prescribed pharmaceutical antifungal). Many drug sensitive individuals find GSE to be much better tolerated than other antifungal preparations and I have several patients in whom this product alone helped control chronic candidiasis when no other medication was tolerated or effective.

In the treatment of intestinal protozoan infections, (Giardia lamblia and Amoeba histolytica) GSE has, in some cases, been more effective than Metronidazole (Flagyl) and other prescription antiprotozoan drugs. These drugs are generally so toxic that they cannot be administered for prolonged periods of time, whereas GSE can be administered for weeks or months; prolonged treatment being essential for the cure of chronic protozoan

*infection....I have had some immunosup-
pressed patients taking the preparation for
over a year with no apparent develoment of
side effects or drug resistance.*

Dr. Jeffrey Bland, America's dean of clinical nutrition,
was also at the conference and he agreed that GSE
combined with a sound nutritional program could help
avoid problems caused by pharmaceutical antibiotics.
And Warren Levin, M.D, one of America's leading
holistic physicians, attested to the effectivenesss of GSE
for treating a broad range of germ induced conditions.
I also learned that the Pasteur Institute of France,
Europe's leading AIDS research center, was (and still is)
studying GSE and its potential for prevention and treatment of communicable diseases. I left the conference
excited about the possibilities GSE offered for my practice.

I returned to my office and, as so often happens to
physicians, a patient soon arrived who would help me
evaluate my new-found information. Dorothy S. to
whom I had administered treatment the previous year,
came to me with complaints about a vaginal infection as
well as a systemic Candida albicans infection that had
begun shortly after taking a ten day course of antibiotics for a bladder infection. Her medical doctor, aware of
the relationship between antibiotics and yeast imbalance, had prescribed Nystatin when signs appeared of

Candida overgrowth in the intestinal tract. However, this pharmaceutical caused Dorothy severe headaches and nausea. Other antifungal drugs were tried but they also caused great distress.

Dorothy was now in my office hoping to find a more natural, less toxic cure for her Candida. I directed her to continue her strict anti-candida diet (see Ch. 6, Treating Candida with GSE) and I gave her Grapefruit Seed Extract liquid concentrate which she was to dilute in water and take three times a day. At her next appointment Dorothy made two very dramatic announcements: that GSE was, "the most horribly bitter concoction" she had ever tasted and that she was "feeling terrific!" (I now suggest taking the liquid concentrate in fruit or vegetable juice to neutralize the bitter taste.)

After two days of initial discomfort (probably from the die-off of the yeast) she awoke feeling clear-headed and energetic for the first time in weeks. Her bloating and headaches were gone, and her stomach no longer rumbled. I continued to monitor Dorothy over the next several weeks. She experienced virtually no side effects from the extract, and after approximately four weeks of use, she required only a small maintenance dose. Dorothy's enthusiasm about her response was equalled only by my own. Though I had recommended other botanically derived remedies to my Candida patients, I had never witnessed such a rapid, complete, and lasting response. It wasn't long before I had another opportunity to test the efficacy of Grapefruit Seed Extract.

Emma L. made an appointment to discuss a disturbing complex of symptoms which began shortly after returning from a camping trip. Although she had no previous digestive problems, Emma now noticed that many foods upset her stomach. She had intermittent bouts of diarrhea and had lost quite a bit of weight. Furthermore she was exhausted most of the time and had a persistent sour taste in her mouth.

A medical doctor had sent her to a local hospital for a stool analysis but the test failed to reveal any of the suspected parasites. She received no recommendation for treatment except to remain on a bland diet, an approach she tried with no success. I told her that many hospitals were not equipped to perform an accurate stool analysis, and that hidden infections often go undetected. I had Emma send a stool sample to Great Smokies Laboratory of Asheville, North Carolina, known for their state of the art approach to stool analysis. Sure enough a parasitic amoeba was discovered! Since GSE had a reputation as an effective antiparasitic, I outlined a program for Emma using GSE as a cornerstone. I was cautiously optimistic because GSE had demonstrated an ability to inhibit the growth of this particular amoeba *en vitro*.

However, laboratory judgements about the effectiveness of an antimicrobial do not always accurately predict the outcome of treatment in a clinical setting. Factors such as correct dosage, absorption, and the ability to tolerate the antimicrobial are not always easy to assess. Furthermore, some parasites burrow deep within the epithelial layers of the intestines and are thus vulnerable to only the most powerful (and toxic) drugs. With these factors in mind, Emma undertook a course of GSE between meals as well as an Aloe vera drink to help cleanse and heal her intestines.

There was no apparent improvement for the first two weeks. In the third week Emma began to notice a subtle but distinct change. She slowly regained much needed weight, her bowel movements were soft but no longer watery, and best of all her energy was returning. In three more weeks, Emma was restored to her old self. A follow-up stool analysis confirmed the success of the treatment.

Not all cases of parasitic infection respond as well to GSE or, for that matter, to any combination of drugs and herbs. Factors that influence successful treatment are:

- Duration of infection
- Virulence of the parasite
- The tendency of parasites to form resistant spores

• The ability of parasites to burrow beneath the surface layers of the intestines (sometimes migrating to deeper tissues such as the liver, spleen, lungs, brain). Most physicians agree that GSE is more effective when administered at the early stages of infestation.

The previous cases illustrate the effectiveness of GSE in the war against yeast and parasites (protozoa), but it is the anti-bacterial nature of GSE that has been most thoroughly documented. One case in particular comes to mind.

In 1992 Dan K., a senior at Boston College, suddenly experienced a bout of ill health which forced him to drop out of school soon after the start of the fall semester. After a prolonged case of what appeared to be a flu, Dan noticed that his energy never fully returned. His digestion was affected and he was experiencing a good deal of pain in several joints.

While in Boston he was seen by several medical specialists. Recurrent intestinal upset and sore throat, joint pain, and blurred vision suggested Lyme's disease, Epstein-Barr virus syndrome, or chronic fatigue syndrome. However these diagnoses were ruled out by extensive laboratory testing. After ten weeks of illness, both Dan and his parents were desperate.

My initial interview revealed that Dan's symptoms began shortly after he had stayed with friends at a college dormitory that he described as less than sanitary. Could he have contracted a parasite or bacteria under those conditions? Because intestinal symptoms were prominent, I thought a stool analysis (by Great Smokies Lab) might once again reveal the culprit. While no parasites were found, a 4+ level (the highest rating) of the bacteria Klebsiella pneumonia was found. For most people the presence of this bacteria seems to cause no outstanding problems, but some do exhibit many of the symptoms that were so disturbing to Dan.

Great Smokies tests the efficacy of both pharmaceutical and herbal products and in this instance, Great Smokies' sensitivity testing clearly showed Grapefruit Seed Extract to be effective against the offending germ. This particular strain of Klebsiella was also sensitive to several pharmaceutical antibiotics. Dan opted for GSE treatment over any of the pharmaceutical antibiotics.

I recommended that Dan use the GSE liquid concentrate in juice three times daily. Given my previous experiences with GSE, I was not surprised when, after ten days, he announced a significant improvement in his health . But he couldn't tolerate the bitter taste of the liquid concentrate so I recommended he switch to the GSE capsules. This improved his compliance and his progress began to accelerate. Within six weeks of his first dose of GSE, Dan's health returned to normal. He eventually returned to college and by attending summer school, graduated in August. Naturally his parents were pleased and also surprised that Dan's condition, which had baffled several medical experts, responded so well to a product derived from grapefruit.

As a practitioner of the natural healing arts, I have always believed that educating my patients is absolutely essential for proper case management. But just as often, my patients teach me.

Charles P., a traveling salesman, had frequent bouts of indigestion—while on the road, the purity of his food was always questionable. He asked me if there was any way to protect himself from germ contamination without taking pharmaceutical antibiotics on a regular basis. I suggested that he use ten to fifteen drops of Grapefruit Seed Extract in juice, after any meal he considered suspect. In the following months he reported that his bouts of severe indigestion were nearly non-existent, thanks to GSE. But he was equally excited about another use he had found for the extract.

Charles suffered from occasional outbreaks of cold sores, caused by the Herpes Symplex 1 virus. Shortly after the start of his last road trip, he experienced a particularly severe outbreak on his lower lip. Scheduled to deliver a speech to potential customers the following day, Charles was desperate. Having no other recourse, he decided to use the GSE by diluting the liquid concentrate with ten parts water which he applied before retiring that night.

The next morning he awoke to feel a slight tingling on his lip. He approached the mirror cautiously but what he saw brought him joy, not dismay. The two cold sores had dried up and shrunk to a fraction of their original size, and the pain he had felt the night before on moderate finger pressure had disappeared.

Now, years later we know from test results that GSE is an effective anti-viral agent in general, and effective for Herpes Symplex 1 in particular. Since it is very astringent (attracts and absorbs moisture), it was no wonder that Charles' cold sore was a mere shadow of its original self, all in a matter of hours.

Since Charles reported his innovative use of GSE, I have recommended it—with excellent results—to many of my patients who are susceptible to cold sores. I am also indebted to Charles because on two occasions I suffered a similar fate, only to experience almost instaneous relief from the extract. One word of caution however: some cold sores can be extremely painful so it is best to start with a very dilute solution of GSE. (Alternative: apply a small amount of GSE powder from a capsule directly to the sore. See under Cold Sores, Ch. 7).

Another little known use for GSE is the treatment of warts. On one of the weekly mountain hikes I take with my friend Marty, he asked me to examine a sizeable bump which had recently developed on his hand. Having lost his sight to glaucoma many years earlier, Marty could only guess at its nature. It was clearly a wart and since warts are most often induced by a virus, I suggested that he try using Grapefruit Seed Extract for a few weeks before resorting to any medical procedures. In this instance, I recommended that he use the extract at full strength, taking care to avoid excessive contact with surrounding skin. I warned him that GSE at full strength would irritate sensitive areas such as lips and eyes.

It was a cold wintry day the next time Marty and I took our hike. After walking for twenty minutes I asked him about his wart. He confessed that he had only used the extract for the first three days and then had become distracted by a demanding schedule. He had forgotten not only about the treatment, but about the wart as well. He removed his glove and felt for the bump. Unable to find it, he kept searching and, slightly confused, felt his other hand.

Only after his thorough examination failed to reveal anything did I take my turn. Sure enough, where last week there had been a sizeable wart, only the faintest flat pink abrasion remained. Needless to say, Marty was thrilled and I was too. A few months later on April 1, Marty received a bill for two hundred dollars for the removal of a wart. When his secretary read it to him he must have developed something much worse than a wart. Then she conveyed to him my best wishes on April Fools Day!

Some types of warts do not respond as well to GSE. Plantar warts, found on the soles of the feet, usually grow inward and may be very resistant to most topical treatment. However, pedunculated warts which have a stalk, can be quite vulnerable to GSE (see under Warts, Ch. 7).

The aforementioned cases represent but a few of the many remarkable results that I have seen with GSE. Furthermore my observations have been confirmed by thousands of physicians nationwide and beyond who have equally dramatic accounts of the efficacy of the extract. It would be unrealistic however to expect that any substance would be universally effective. Because of misdiagnosis, resistant or inaccessible germs, lack of patient compliance, or inability to tolerate the extract, I have often had to recommend other modalities.

I believe that there are cases where there is no recourse but a pharmaceutical antibiotic. It is a challenge to the physician to recognize such a situation. To "err on the side of caution" by indiscriminately prescribing antibiotics is simply bad medicine but to stubbornly adhere to an "holistic" approach can be just as dangerous. If infection is suspected, it is necessary to consult a trained professional. And it should also be remembered that antimicrobial agents are only a stop-gap measure. The strengthening and support of the immune system should be the highest priority of patient and physician alike.

While the experiences of my patients convinced me that GSE was a potent and effective germ inhibitor it was, quite naturally, my own experience with the extract that has left an indelible impression on me.

Six months after I began recommending GSE to my patients, I attended a farewell party for a friend of mine at a smoke-filled bar. Because of my sensitivity to cigarette smoke, I wasn't surprised to find that I had a scratchy throat the next day. In the past, a sore throat from secondary smoke (which weakens my immune system) would certainly have led to several days of uncomfortable cold and sinus symptoms. I decided to do exactly what I would suggest to my patients—gargle with a dilute solution of GSE. I put twenty drops of the concentrate into six ounces of water and gargled with this rather bitter solution. Then I immediately swallowed a similar amount of GSE. The taste wasn't pleasant but the results were. Within a few minutes I could swallow with virtually no pain. To reinforce the results I repeated the treatment but this time gargling with GSE powder. The throat irritation was gone and even more exciting was the fact that my anticipated sinus condition never developed. Apparently the opportunistic germs, that usually attack when my tissue undergoes the shock of cigarette allergy, were stopped dead in their tracks.

Only three weeks later I had another opportunity to save myself from considerable discomfort. I was attending a conference on the West Coast and though I had managed to maintain a fairly good diet while traveling, one of the meals finally got to me. By the time I returned to my hotel room I began to experience all of the symptoms caused by contaminated food. I had experienced those symptoms before so I didn't have much hope that I'd be able to attend a workshop I was particularly interested in, scheduled for the following day. As my nausea mounted and the rumbling in my stomach became more ominous I took a double dose of GSE liquid concentrate in orange juice. I repeated this fifteen minutes later and stumbled to bed to wait out a miserable evening. The next morning I was startled by the wake-up call. I had slept through the night and on rising felt altogether fine except for a small area of soreness in my lower abdomen. I felt a little weak that day but I was able to attend the workshop.

Now, whenever I travel, I always carry GSE. And at home it is one of the most important components of my first-aid kit. Many of my patients feel the same way about GSE.

6

TREATING CANDIDA WITH GRAPEFRUIT SEED EXTRACT

MANY HOLISTIC PHYSICIANS, myself included, consider *Candida albicans* one of the greatest health challenges to people of the industrialized nations. The broad spectrum, antifungal properties of GSE have made it an important part of successful anti-Candida programs—a fact which has linked the names Candida and Grapefruit Seed Extract. With the help of GSE, thousands of individuals have overcome the multiple effects of Candida.

Candida albicans is a prime example of an opportunistic pathogen (disease causing agent). Its presence in the digestive tract and in the urogenital tract is, of itself, not remarkable—nearly every human harbors small amounts of this ubiquitous germ. The toxins that Candida produces are only mildly irritating as long as their numbers are in check. Rarely are high fevers, elevated white blood cell counts, severe diarrhea, etc. associated with Candida, as might be the case with so many other pathogens. However, when the opportunity presents itself, the yeast can begin to grow at an alarming rate. And as Candida grows, so does the concentration of its toxins; eventually even the most stalwart individuals will begin to suffer from the effects of yeast imbalance.

Candida is usually found in the small and large intestines and the urogenital tract (of men and women) where it competes for food and attachment sites with other microorganisms. Many researchers now believe that certain forms of the yeast can travel through the blood and eventually inhabit any organ of the body. Once Candida overgrowth takes hold, the potential for adverse effects is enormous: fatigue, indigestion, flatulence, constipation, diarrhea, depression, anxiety, and a diminished libido are the most common effects: others include carbohydrate and alcohol cravings, frequent bladder and ear infections, various skin afflictions (acne, eczema) and reactions to perfume, cleansing agents, gasoline fumes, etc. For women, frequent vaginal infections and menstrually related symptoms signal the possibility that Candida is out of control.

The Genesis of Candida

How does an overgrowth of yeast come about? Studies have shown that the typical human digestive tract is inhabited by well over one thousand varieties of fungal, bacterial, viral, and protozoan species. The competition within this ecological environment is fierce: food and attachment sites are limited—only the fittest survive.

It is estimated that the microorganisms inhabiting the digestive tract of the average adult number in the hundreds of trillions. In fact, there are many times the number of such microorganisms than there are body cells. Most of the microbes belong to species that neither help nor hurt us. This relationship between host and visitor is called *commensuralism*. Other species of microorganisms that perform scores of life-sustaining tasks are absolutely essential for our well-being. These are the *symbiots*: Lactobacillus acidophilus and Bifidobacterium bifidus belong to this group. A third class of microbes is considered parasitic because it grows at the expense of the host, often leading to illness and even death. The proportional balance of microbes residing within each individual depends on many factors: exposure to various microbes, age, diet, nutritional status, emotional stress, antibiotic-use (from drugs and food) and the general functioning of the immune system.

Given these (and other) factors, we can expect to find a different mix of microorganisms not only from one individual to another, but also from one geographical area to another. For example, the protozoa *Entamoeba histolytica*, is considered endemic in India and Pakistan. But the indigenous population has adapted itself to that amoeba which, though it may weaken them somewhat, is not as pathogenic as it is to an American tourist, for example, who is encountering it for the first time. Although mainstream medicine has perceived the endemic nature of *E. histolytica* in India, it has failed to recognize that people of the industrialized West have biologically selected out *Candida albicans* as one of our endemic species. And while symptoms associated with Candida imbalance are not as dramatic as those associated with certain amoebas, the insidious development of a Candida imbalance can lead to years of suffering, the cause of which often remains undiagnosed by conventional medical practice.

THE PROLIFERATION OF CANDIDA

Why is Candida so common in the digestive tracts of people living in the industrialized nations? Ironically, most of the blame lies in our technology and the way we use and abuse it. Some of the practices that create a susceptibility to systemic Candida overgrowth are:

- Excessive use of pharmaceutical antibiotics
- Ingestion of meat and poultry treated with antibiotics
- Chlorination of drinking water
- Exposure to pesticides, herbicides, chemicals, toxic metals (lead, mercury)
- Hormonal treatment (including birth control pills and cortisone products)
- Poor diet (insufficient essential nutrients; excessive use of sugar, carbohydrates, alcohol)

Beneficial bacteria such as Lactobacillus and Bifidobacterium which secrete powerful antifungal enzymes that support the digestive and urogenital tracts are destroyed by pharmaceutical antibiotics, chlorine, and toxins found in food and drink. Once the health of our beneficial bacteria is compromised, an ecological niche opens up that is rapidly filled by other microorganisms, Candida among them. Because western diets are so rich in carbohydrates (sugars and starches), Candida and other carbohydrate-loving yeasts find the digestive tract an ideal environment.

While primary Candida imbalance inflicts great stress upon the immune system, it often happens that Candida is a secondary result of a longstanding immune dysfunction. AIDS, cancer, and chronic fatigue patients are always at risk of Candida imbalance. Their treatment must take into account the likelihood of additional stress from yeast.

Many of the pharmaceutical drugs that are used to fight Candida have proven quite toxic, especially to the liver. But there is good news too. According to worldwide reports from holistic physicians and thousands of their patients, GSE is one of the best non-toxic remedies for Candida. Dr. Jay Gordon, a highly respected pediatrician practicing in California states:

> *I have been in private practice for sixteen years... I discovered GSE about five years ago. We pediatricians treat a lot of oral and cutaneous yeast infections (the latter primarily in the diaper area of infants) and are often frustrated at the difficulty we have in clearing up these common and annoying problems. I now recommend GSE at least three to four times every day to my patients and the response is uniformly positive...GSE is an excellent formulation which I have found to be completely safe for even the youngest babies in my practice.*

Treating Candida with GSE

For chronic cases of Candida imbalance, it is best to prepare for GSE therapy by performing a one week cleansing diet. Such a diet curtails starchy, sugar-rich foods and eliminates fermented foods, coffee, cigarettes, and alcohol; it calls for the following (approximate) proportions:

- 65% high fiber, low starch vegetables (broccoli, celery, radish, asparagus, etc.—steamed or raw)
- 20% high protein foods (fish, fowl [free of antibiotics], nuts, seeds, eggs, tofu, etc.)
- 10% complex carbohydrates (rice, beans, millet, amaranth, quinoa, buckwheat)
- 5% fruit (papaya, pineapple, grapefruit, and all types of berries)

Such a diet reduces the unpleasant effects (known as the "Herxheimer reaction" after the doctor who described it) caused by the release of toxins when pathogenic microbes 'die-off.' A Herxheimer reaction may temporarily cause increased fatigue, nausea, headache, etc. These reactions are common but usually occur only in the first few weeks of treatment.

For optimum results I also recommend that my patients consume six to eight capsules per day of a high potency, high quality probiotic containing Lactobacillus, Bifidobacterium, etc. Garlic and Aloe vera assist the detoxification process. If a Candida imbalance is not chronic but has been brought on by a recently prescribed course of antibiotics, the above diet and the GSE treatment can begin simultaneously and continue for at least three to four weeks.

Treatment

GSE should be taken between meals. If irritating to the digestive tract, it may be taken with meals or in powder form (capsule). Dosages given are for a person of approximately 150 lbs.; adjust dosage according to weight.

Days 1–3: ten drops (50/50 dilution, see page 124) twice daily in vegetable or diluted fruit juice (or one 125 mg. capsule twice daily)

Days 4–10: fifteen drops twice daily (or one capsule three times daily)

Days 11-28: fifteen drops three times daily (or two capsules two to three times daily)

Some people will show satisfactory improvement on the lower doses and therefore not require an increase; on the other hand, some resistant cases may require a slightly higher dose than given above. The schedule may also be modified: for some, the twenty-eight day course may prove unnecessary—two to three weeks may suffice. Once satisfactory improvement is noted, gradually reduce the GSE dosage; if symptoms reappear, a return to a higher dose may be required. A four week treatment may not be sufficient—longstanding chronic cases may require four to six *months* of constant vigilance.

Vaginal yeast infection

Many holistic physicians believe that an imbalance in the vaginal microflora is often indicative of a similiar imbalance in the intestinal tract. Therefore, for recurrent vaginal yeast infections, a complete, systemic anti-Candida program is usually required. However, certain isolated instances of vaginal yeast imbalance may be treated locally without resorting to a systemic program.

Note: Before beginning any treatment for vaginal infection, a diagnosis by a qualified practitioner is necessary in order to establish whether or not the perceived symptoms are in fact being caused by Candida. The possibility of reinfection by transmission from a sexual partner must also be considered if a cure is to be permanent.

Treatment

Vaginal rinse: add sixteen drops of GSE to sixteen ounces of room temperature water (use only filtered, distilled, or boiled water) and shake well in a closed jar.

Douche once daily for three days. (For greater retention of the solution, douche in a reclining position.) Repeat every fifth day thereafter.

Caution: If severe vaginal irritation occurs, reduce mixture to five drops per pint of water. Discontinue if irritation persists. Do not douche if pregnant or menstruating unless advised by a physician.

Most chronic Candida problems, whether systemic or localized, are related to certain life-style habits. Therefore GSE should be considered an adjunct to the changes required for permanent resolution of the problem. To conclude this chapter I offer a condensed version of my Ten Step Program for Controlling Candida.

1. Be Informed: Read at least one book on Candida. (see suggested reading list). Seek a qualified practitioner who can direct your program but do not depend solely on his or her expertise—talk to others who have successfully overcome Candida.

2. Starve the yeast: Candida thrives on carbohydrates: drastically reduce all foods high in starch and sugars.

3. Avoid yeast products and fermented foods: Baker's and brewer's yeast, wine, vinegar (apple cider vinegar may be tolerated), tempeh, and tamari are potential trouble-makers.

4. Use non-toxic antifungals: Botanically derived antifungals are preferred because they do not add to the body's toxic load. GSE's broad spectrum capabilities detoxify the system not only from Candida but also from other yeasts and bacteria which accompany Candida. GSE is also effective with other herbal antifungals such as Pao' D' arco, garlic, and goldenseal. (Consume antifungals between meals.)

5. **Restore the beneficial bacteria:** Probiotics, particularly Lactobacillus acidopohilus and Bifidobacterium bifidus help reestablish the normal intestinal flora. This phase of the treatment will, in the long run, protect against reinfection. (Consume probiotics with meals.)

6. **Support the beneficial bacteria:** These helpful symbiots thrive in the presence of foods rich in fiber and chlorophyll. Fructo-oligo-saccharides (F.O.S.) is a type of sugar (found in the Jerusalem artichoke) which can dramatically increase the growth rate of beneficial bacteria, especially Bifidobacterium, an organism essential for a healthy digestive tract. F.O.S. cannot be metabolized by Candida, nor does it significantly raise the blood sugar.

7. **Detoxify:** Eliminate (or greatly reduce) coffee, alcohol, food with chemical additives, and drugs. Aloe vera, Bentonite clay, and psyllium seeds can accelerate the detoxification process. Drink at least 6-8 glasses of *non-chlorinated* water daily.

8. **Support the immune system:** Reduce emotional and chemical stress. Supplement your diet with the

proper vitamins, minerals and antioxidants (Vitamins A, E, C, lipoic acid, glutathione, selenium, pycnogenol, Coenzyme Q10, etc.) which are essential for reversing damage done to the immune system.

9. Be observant: Write down all of your symptoms before starting the program and grade them on a scale of 1–10 according to how they affect you. Compare those observations to how you feel four, six, and eight weeks later. You will have good days and not-so-good days so when you feel poorly, instead of cursing the darkness, light a candle of understanding: Did you go off the diet? Were you in a smoke-filled room? Did you clean out a moldy basement? Women: note where you are in your menstrual cycle; record your observations—you will learn more about how your body works and why sometimes it does not.

10. Persist: A restoration of the internal environment does not happen overnight—this program takes time. It is a starting point, a general guide that can be adapted to your own needs. Once you feel an improvement, avoid the temptation to revert to former habits.

7

TREATING
COMMON
HEALTH
PROBLEMS
WITH
GRAPEFRUIT
SEED EXTRACT

I N MY RESEARCH OF GSE I have gathered information from hundreds of physicians and their patients. This, as well as my own experience, both as physician and consumer, has enabled me to appreciate the great versatility of this substance. This chapter presents some common conditions of ill health for which the properties of GSE have come to be held in the highest regard.

The suggested uses presented here are based on a fifty/fifty mix of 'Standardized Extract' and vegetable glycerine (see explanation following Table 1, Ch. 2). Some manufacturers follow the commendable practice of providing a small instructional brochure with each bottle. At present there are no official standards of potency for the various GSE liquid concentrates currently available so if you are unsure about the potency of a particular product, call the manufacturer for clarification. Do not expect these companies to offer diagnosis or treatment protocols.

GSE is also available in dry form as tablets and capsules; one need only consult the product label for milligram counts per tablet or capsule. Some companies list milligram counts per <u>two</u> or more capsules on their labels: this must be accounted for when calculating proper dosage.

A typical capsule of GSE contains between 100mg and 125mg (the strength may be less if the GSE is combined with other herbs). One capsule is approximately equal to ten drops of the aforementioned fifty/fifty liquid concentrate. Therefore a recommendation of four capsules per day could be substituted, for certain applications, by 40 drops of liquid concentrate (fifty percent solution) and vice versa.

Note: The suggested uses given here are not to be construed as a diagnosis or as a recomendation for the treatment of any condition of ill health. Rather it is provided for research purposes only. See author's advisory at the beginning of this book.

ACNE

Acne may develop when the skin is unable to mount an effective defense against microbes, especially bacteria. It often appears in adolescents due to hormonal changes and sometimes remains as a lifelong affliction.

Its incidence is greater in patients with fungal imbalance (e.g., Candida). It may also be caused by allergies to certain foods (wheat, milk, chocolate, etc,) and by bacterial growth in skin pores due to improper hygiene. GSE inhibits this bacterial growth and its astringency dries up glandular secretions (sebum) thus reducing breeding opportunities for bacteria.

Treatment

External: Five drops of GSE liquid concentrate added to each application of your regular liquid cleanser creates a superior cleansing solution. Avoid contact with the eyes. For convenience, GSE concentrate may be added to a bottle of cleanser in a concentration of one to three percent GSE. A greater concentration is likely to dry the skin (especially the face) if used regularly.

Internal: A chronic condition may require internal cleansing. Ten–fifteen drops of GSE (diluted in juice), three times daily.

AIDS

No claim can be made that GSE will cure AIDS, but an increasing number of HIV positive people are beginning to use it to defend themselves against fungi, bacteria, viruses or parasites—secondary infections common in those suffering from the disease. Candida, for example, is one of the most troubling of these infections. (See Ch. 6, Treating Candida with GSE.)

When used as a gargle, GSE can relieve a sore throat (see under Sore Throat) and perhaps reduce the need for pharmaceutical antibiotics. Since AIDS patients are highly susceptible to parasites such as Amoeba, Giardia, and Cryptosporidium, GSE can help maintain health by reducing the number of these potentially lethal invaders.

A recent government study has indicated that a large percentage of municipal water systems harbor parasites such as Cryptosporidium, which appears to survive chlorination. Since GSE may be many times stronger than chlorine in its ability to control certain organisms, it may prove to be a viable alternative for protecting immune deficient individuals from Cryptosporidium.

Many HIV positive people are adding GSE to water and to soak their fruit, vegetables, fish, meat, and poultry in dilute solutions of GSE for ten to fifteen minutes (followed by thorough rinsing). This practice reduces the risk of E. coli and Salmonella which in small amounts may be harmless to a healthy immune system but are quite dangerous to the AIDS patient.

Since those with AIDS are susceptible to many skin, ear, throat, rectal, and vaginal infections, GSE can be used for these applications as well. (See under specific condition and Ch. 10, Household and Other Uses for GSE.)

Treatment

The form and amount of GSE required naturally depends on the intended purpose. Since people with AIDS are often sensitive to new substances, it is best to begin with a reduced dosage when used internally. For topical uses as well as household ones, typical amounts as listed under each application can be used.

ARTHRITIS

Researchers have long postulated that some forms of arthritis, especially rheumatoid arthritis, may be related to bacterial strep infection. New evidence suggests that several other bacteria may also be implicated, two of which are *Proteus vulgaris* and *Klebsiella pneumonia*, both frequently found in the digestive tract.

According to the research, our immune systems produce antibodies to neutralize antigens produced by these bacteria. These antibody-antigen complexes may be absorbed by the intestinal lining and thus enter the bloodstream. In most instances the body handles the antigen-antibody complexes through the liver, kidney, and lymphatic detoxification mechanisms. However, in some individuals, the complex can trigger a reaction leading to serious complications.

With Klebsiella pneumonia, this reaction usually occurs in the spinal column. A debilitating condition known as *ankylosing spodolytis* may ensue and cause vertebral segments of the spinal column to fuse into a ramrod type structure resulting in a devastating loss of spinal flexibility.

In the case of Proteus vulgaris complexes, inflammatory responses can occur in any joint resulting in swelling, pain, and deformity, the telltale signs of rheumatoid arthritis. As research goes forward, we can expect that other microbes responsible for joint inflammation will be identified. And they will not be limited to bacterial species; already arthritic reactions have been attributed to various fungal, viral and parasitic strains.

Some patients have noticed that their arthritic symptoms were either temporarily or permanently improved when treated with pharmaceutical antibiotics for conditions *other* than arthritis. This led to some of the original research on the arthritis/microbe connection. I have received numerous reports stating that individuals using GSE on a regular basis for Candida, dysentery etc., have noticed a significant improvement in their arthritic conditions. While the relief from arthritis may have been brought about by the reduction of the Candida syndrome, it is equally likely that the reduction in the population of allergy inducing bacteria was also responsible for the improvement.

Treatment

Use ten to fifteen drops of GSE liquid concentrate (mixed in juice) three to four times per day (or two capsules three times per day) between meals. If GSE is relevent to the condition, improvement is likely to occur in four to eight weeks. It is also helpful to take probiotic cultures (Acidophilus, etc) with meals as part of the protocol to reduce the risk of recontamination with the offending germ once the GSE is discontinued. When improvement is noted, continue to use GSE at half the recommended dose for several more weeks to reduce the risk of reoccurence.

Note: While microbes may account for many cases of arthritis, acute episodes or arthritic flare-ups often represent inflammation brought on by an allergic response to food, dust, mold, or chemicals. Nutritional deficiencies may also lead to arthritis.

ATHLETE'S FOOT

This condition occurs when the skin is unable to ward off fungal overgrowth (opportunistic fungi are always present). Since fungi thrive in warm, dark, moist places, it is necessary to keep the feet dry and exposed to moderate amounts of sunlight. Wear cotton socks and never wear wet shoes or sneakers. Resistant cases may need to be treated systemically for yeast imbalance (see Ch. 6, Treating Candida with GSE) Commercially available foot powders with GSE (some products contain additional antifungal substances) work remarkably well.

Treatment

Apply a footpowder containing approximately five to ten percent GSE powder to the feet twice daily. Proper hygiene will prevent reinfection. Also recommended: soak socks in water containing a small amount of GSE liquid concentrate before laundering (fungi often survive regular wash cycles).

BELCHING (See FLATULENCE)

BODY ODOR

GSE's extraordinary ability to control germs makes it an effective deodorant and its astringent quality provides a mild anti-perspirant action.

Treatment

In a spray bottle, mix one-half ounce of GSE with ten ounces of water. Calendula and/or Arnica tincture may be added to the mix. Spray under arms, on feet, etc. as needed. Avoid contact with the eyes.

CANDIDA

(See Ch. 6, Treating Candida with GSE)

CHRONIC FATIGUE SYNDROME (CFIDS)

This is one of the most puzzling and devastating of conditions. It now appears that CFIDS is caused by any number of biochemical, microbial, or nutritional factors which have a disorganizing effect on the immune system. Patients display many debilitating symptoms, the most common being chronic exhaustion, aching muscles, depression, sleep disorders, chemical sensitivities, and heightened susceptibility to viral, bacterial, and fungal infections.

Patients with CFIDS, like those with AIDS and Lymes's disease, are frequently prescribed pharmaceutical antibiotics for transient infections which may further weaken their immunity. In this regard GSE may offer a safe alternative.

Treatment See under specific conditions.

Caution: CFIDS patients frequently experience a burning sensation in their diaphragm and upper stomach area. For this reason, GSE powder may be better tolerated (for internal use) than the liquid concentrate. For internal use, patients with gastric upset should begin with no more than one capsule twice daily and gradually increase to the desired level. If gastric irritation increases, reduce to lower levels and take GSE with at least 16 ounces of water. If this treatment fails to reduce stomach distress, discontinue GSE.

Colds/Flus

Colds and flus are caused by several viral strains and are notoriously resistant to pharmaceutical antibiotics. GSE, which gives optimum results (as many holistic physicians have discovered) when used in combination with immune supportive herbs such as Echinacea, Gold-enseal, and Astragalus, has provided much needed relief to cold and flu sufferers. When an intestinal flu strikes, causing abdominal pain and diarrhea, GSE can hasten recovery by directly attacking the virus in the digestive tract.

Treatment

At the first sign of a cold or flu take fifteen drops of GSE (or two capsules) mixed in juice, three times daily. As an alternative, add fifty drops of GSE to one quart of fruit or vegetable juice and sip throughout the day. Combinations of GSE with the above mentioned herbs are available; use as recommended by a physician.

COLD SORES

These blister-like lesions, caused by the *Herpes simplex 1* virus, usually appear on the face and lips but may appear anywhere on the skin. Genital herpes is thought to be caused by a variant, *Herpes simplex II*, but some researchers now speculate that the same virus may be responsible for both conditions.

The Herpes virus is thought to reside in most individuals but for those who are susceptible, certain conditions of physical, emotional, or nutritional stress bring on a full-blown attack that causes pain and embarrassment. GSE, with its antiviral and astringent properties, can often combat this condition by inactivating the virus and drying up the lesion, sometimes in a matter of hours.

Treatment

Thoroughly mix five drops of GSE with fifty drops of vegetable glycerine (available in health food and drug stores). Apply with a cotton swab two or three times daily. If lesion is especially raw, use only one or two drops of GSE to fifty drops of glycerine. If, on the other hand no irritation occurs with the original mix, you can increase the potency by adding several drops of GSE (mix well). Alternative: Mix one part GSE powder (from capsule) with three parts corn or rice flour. Add a few drops of water to make a paste and apply to the lesion. If burning or irritation occurs remove immediately and add more flour to reduce the potency of the GSE.

Cuts/Wounds

GSE's powerful germ fighting ability makes it an ideal antiseptic alternative. Products which use isopropyl alcohol and iodine are also effective germ killers but their toxic nature may retard the growth of granulation tissue which is required to heal a wound. GSE, on the other hand, appears to encourage the process of healing. Perhaps due in part to its astringency and its citrus origins, healing time is often remarkably short with the proper use of GSE.

Keep a solution of GSE on hand for emergencies: Thoroughly mix one-half ounce GSE with eight ounces of distilled water. Pour solution into a clean spray bottle.

Note: Excellent results have been reported by adding a small amount of liquid herbal extract such as Echinacea, Goldenseal, Calendula (marigold), or Plantago major (Plantain) to the GSE solution.

Treatment

Spray GSE solution (as above) liberally over the affected area once every few minutes while performing other standard first aid procedures. If the wound is deep or widespread a highly dilute mixture of GSE is indicated. In such cases begin with less than one-quarter teaspoon GSE in ten ounces of water. More GSE can be gradually added to the mixture if no irritation is noted.

Caution: In case of severe wound or burn, see a licensed physician immediately. Do not apply GSE as further irritation is likely to occur.

DANDRUFF

According to dermatologists, dandruff is most often caused by an inflammatory reaction to an overgrowth of scalp fungus which causes itching and scaling. In cases where skin fungus is the cause, good results may be obtained by adding a few drops of GSE to one's regular shampoo. It should be noted however, that excessive washing of the hair removes natural oils that protect the scalp from fungi. In difficult cases, internal treatment for yeast imbalance may be necessary (see Ch. 6, Treating Candida with GSE).

Treatment

Add ten drops of GSE liquid concentrate to each application of shampoo. Mix thoroughly before applying to the scalp. Wait three to five minutes before rinsing.

Avoid contact with the eyes. If contact occurs, rinse thoroughly with water.

DIAPER RASH

This all too common problem is usually caused by allergic reactions to the diaper material or to food residues in the urine and/or feces. Allowing a child to remain wet for a prolonged period of time is a guarantee that a fungal overgrowth will produce a diaper rash. If a microorganism is causing the rash, GSE powder may prove effective.

Treatment

Mix thoroughly one part GSE powder, one part slippery elm powder (available at many health food stores) and fifteen parts finely milled rice, corn, or cassava root flour (tapioca). Apply this mixture twice daily to the affected area. Discontinue if treatment aggravates condition. As an alternative, try a GSE footpowder.

Note: avoid talc products; they may cause irritation and if inhaled, may be fatal to children.

In persistant cases internal treatment may be necessary and should be given only under the supervision of a professional health care provider. A probiotic containing Bifidobacterium bifidus and Acidophilus added to the infant's food can help rebalance the intestinal flora. GSE powder taken orally in appropriate amounts may also be beneficial.

Diarrhea

This condition, like so many, has a variety of causes. If it is caused by a bacteria, fungus, or virus, a few doses of GSE may be all that is needed. Parasitic dysentery (*Amoebiasis, Giardiasis, etc.*) may be more stubborn and require weeks of treatment with GSE and other herbs (some cases may require pharmaceutical drugs). In all cases of parasitic infection it is important to begin treatment with a licensed practitioner as soon as possible. (See also Parasitic Infection.)

Treatment

Use fifteen to twenty drops of GSE (or two capsules) diluted in juice every four hours up to sixty drops per day. Always supplement with probiotics to replace beneficial bacteria lost in the watery stool. For parasites, a higher dosage may be required: consult a qualified physician.

EARACHE (Otitis media)

This ailment accounts for more visits to the pediatrician's office than any other. Adults, especially those who swim, are also susceptible. Commercially available eardrops which contain a miniscule amount of GSE offer excellent symptomatic relief. They are likely to contain synergystic herbal extracts as well. Additional treatement may be recommended by a qualified physcian.

Treatment

Use one to three drops of a commercially prepared GSE ear product twice daily.

Caution: Use only products formulated specifically for the ear. Do not use GSE liquid concentrate directly in the ear. In the event of such contact, flush with copious amounts of water.

EYE PROBLEMS

When a bacteria or a virus infects the eyes, it causes redness and inflammation. Pinkeye (conjunctivitis) is usually self-limiting but can easily be passed on to family members. While some doctors have reported benefits from using a solution of *one* drop of GSE in a full ounce of distilled water (thoroughly shaken), the use of GSE for eye problems is still under investigation and therefore *cannot* be recommended due to the acidic nature of GSE. It definitely should not be considered as a remedy for children since their eyes are even more sensitive than adult's eyes. However, the addition of GSE to a liquid hand soap and to laundry detergent may prevent the spread of the disease to other family members.

Preventing the Spread of Conjunctivitis

Prepare a three percent solution of GSE in liquid soap. All family members should wash their hands regularly with the soap whether or not they show symptoms of conjunctivitis. Before washing towels, soak them for fifteen minutes in a pail of water to which one hundred drops of GSE liquid concentrate has been added.

FLATULENCE

Gas in the digestive tract is usually caused by the fermention of carbohydrates by microorganisms: yeast (Candida), bacteria, and some parasites are often involved. For most people flatulence is merely embarrassing, but for some it can be painful. Excess gas bloats the abdomen, a serious medical condition that warrants thorough screening for food allergies and/or intolerances.

If the flatulence is caused by excessive yeast or bacteria it can usually be brought under control in a few days with GSE. But if parasites are the cause, a quick resolution is less likely.

Treatment

Use ten to twenty drops of GSE (one or two capsules) in juice three times daily before or after meals. An appropriate probiotic and digestive enzymes taken before meals often proves helpful. If symptoms persist, consult a physician.

FOOD CONTAMINATION/FOOD POISONING
(see DIARRHEA)

GUMS (gingivitis)

Inflammation of the gums (gingivitis) is often caused by bacteria, though fungi and viruses may also be involved. A buildup of plaque indicates the presence of certain bacteria that bind minerals and deposit them on the gums. Excessive plaque causes gums to recede and leads to a loss of teeth. Gingivitis can also result from nutritional deficiencies (typically Vitamins A and C).

GSE is also effective for treating the small ulcers that appear so often on the gums and inside the lips. Some consumers have reported immediate relief upon applying a solution of five drops GSE mixed thoroughly into fifty drops of vegetable glycerine. GSE's extraordinary cleansing ability has been put to good use in oral care products such as a toothpaste, mouth wash, and gum cleanser.

Treatment

General gum care: dilute five to ten drops of GSE in six to eight ounces of water; swish in mouth then rinse thoroughly. (To avoid the bitter taste, pour the powdered contents of one capsule into six to eight ounces of water; mix thoroughly.)

Caution: Do not apply GSE full strength directly on the gums or teeth as it may eventually erode the protective enamel.

The addition of a few drops of GSE to the reservoir of hydraulic teeth cleaning devices cleans both the gums and the reservoir and tubing of the device (see Ch. 10, Household Uses.).

IMPETIGO

Impetigo is a skin infection (most often affecting children) which causes an itchy rash-like outbreak on the face or elsewhere on the body. It is distinguished by a clear to yellow discharge of pus which keeps the affected area wet. Impetigo is usually caused by bacteria, in particular *Group A beta hemolytic streptococcus.* More recently however, Staphylococcus aureus has been implicated in many cases of impetigo. GSE's ability to combat the above mentioned germs makes it a good choice for treating Impetigo.

Treatment

Mix one-half ounce GSE liquid concentrate in five ounces of water; apply to infected area several times daily. Excellent results have been reported by those who have added one-half ounce extract of *Calendula officianlis* (marigold) to the solution. Impetigo should be taken seriously; consult a physician. In certain instances a pharmaceutical prescription may be necessary.

Recurrent episodes of impetigo can be avoided by careful attention to hygiene. Hands and face may be washed with cleansers that contain one to three percent GSE. A one to three percent spray solution of GSE can be used after shaving, on mosquito bites (when scratching is likely), and after handling contaminated articles, etc. One teaspoon of GSE added to the wash cycle will help decontaminate shared towels, linens, etc.

Jock itch

Rashes in the groin and upper thigh areas are most often caused by a fungal overgrowth. This is common in those who are prone to sweating, such as athletes (hence the name *Jock Itch*).

Treatment:

Apply a foot or body powder containing five to ten percent GSE to the affected area twice daily. Jock itch may represent a reduced ability to ward off fungus and thus may require a comprehensive systemic program. (See Ch. 6, Treating Candida with GSE).

LIPS

Cracks and sores on the lips are often healed rapidly with GSE. Cracks in the corners of the mouth (*Angular stomatitis*) may be a result of a vitamin B-2 (riboflavin) deficiency. In such cases, vitamin therapy is indicated.

Treatment (see COLD SORES)

LYME'S DESEASE

The devastating symptoms of this tic borne disease are caused by a spiral-shaped bacterium (spirochete) related to the bacterium which causes syphilis. Patients with Lyme's disease exhibit many of the same symptoms as those with Chronic Fatigue Syndrome with the addition of severe joint swelling and pain.

Some people diagnosed with Lyme's disease have reported dramatic improvement in their symptoms and blood tests with the use of GSE, but it is premature to suggest that GSE works directly against the spirochete. Most of those suffering from Lyme's have been treated with a long-term program of pharmaceutical antibiotics which more often than not leaves the patient with a significant yeast imbalance—Candida. The benefits of GSE may well be in combating such secondary infections.

Treatment:

Since the direct treatment of Lyme's disease with GSE is still under investigation no recommendation can be made at this time. (For the treatment of ensuing Candida imbalance see Ch. 6, "Treating Candida with GSE.")

NAILS

Deformed, discolored, soft or brittle nails are most often caused by fungi that live, and, under certain conditions, thrive underneath the nail. Eventually the nail bed and growth of the nail itself is compromised. Bacteria can also make their way underneath the nails and cause a chronic problem that is not only unattractive, but often painful as well. These fungi and bacteria frequently affect gardeners, body workers, beauticians, dishwashers, and athletes; diabetics and the elderly are the most susceptible.

GSE's broad-spectrum antimicrobial action works well for both treatment and prevention of nail disease. If a fungus is the offending germ, treatment for an internal yeast imbalance may be necessary.

Treatment

For maximum penetration, mix one-half ounce GSE liquid concentrate with five ounces of 80 proof grain alcohol or vodka. Apply under/on the nail with an eye dropper two or three times per day. For better results, scrub gently with a soft nail brush with each application. Because this is a particularly resistant condition, several months of regular use may be necessary.

Prevention: After gardening or other activities which might bring contact with germs, apply aforementioned solution under/on the nail. If one or two nails are already infected, apply the antifungal solution to neighboring nails two or three times per week to prevent the spread of infection.

Nausea

When nausea and/or vomiting is caused by a flu or by germ contaminated water, it is often helpful to regurgitate the stomach contents in order to avoid contaminating the lower digestive tract. Once liquid can be retained, GSE can play an important part in hastening recovery.

Treatment

Add fifty drops of GSE to one quart of diluted juice; sip in small amounts as tolerated.

Parasitic Infection

A parasite is an organism that derives its sustenance from an organism of another species, called the host. While bacteria, fungi, and viruses might technically fall into this category, a parasite is more specifically defined as an animal species with the potential to cause disease or dysfunction. Parasites may be quite large; tape worms, found in the digestive tract, have been known to exceed twenty feet in length. Although parasites are normally found in the digestive tract, they may also infect the lungs, liver, brain and almost any organ of the body.

Certainly the greatest number of parasitic conditions are caused by microscopic, single-celled animals: *Amoeba, Giardia, Trichomonas, Blastocystis hominis,* and *Cryptosporidium* are among the thousands of invaders that represent one of the greatest challenges to physicians of every persuasion. Parasites most often enter the body through the mouth and soon thereafter establish a colony in the digestive tract. The lower intestinal tract seems the most hospitable to these creatures whose infestation may cause watery stools, abdominal pain, gassiness, bloating, fatigue, and weight loss.

The various immune complexes, enzymes, white blood cells, etc. which abound in the digestive tract make life difficult for parasites. To avoid these defenses, they may burrow into the walls (lumen) of the digestive tract and eventually penetrate further into the body. As they sequester themselves, they become more difficult to treat. Therefore it is important to begin treatment as soon after infection as possible. Of course it is far better to practice prevention; in both arenas, GSE can play an important role.

Prevention: GSE is a great traveling companion whether you're heading for an exotic corner of the world or eating in a local restaurant of dubious hygiene. If you have eaten or drunk something you suspect may be contaminated, take twenty to thirty drops of GSE liquid concentrate in juice (or three capsules). You can repeat this every two hours for at least three doses.

Wilderness streams, as pristine as they might appear, are often contaminated by Giardia and other parasites from wild animals. Avoid drinking such water but if necessary it can be treated with ten drops of GSE per six ounces of water; let stand fifteen minutes (add flavoring to reduce bitter taste).

Caution: Despite the effectiveness of GSE against many forms of parasites, one should never suspend normal sanitary precautions. Better to avoid contact than to trust that GSE, or any other anti-parasitic, will save the day.

If a parasitic infection is suspected consult a licensed physician as soon as possible for proper identification of the offending germ. The amount of GSE recommended may be three to four times that used for bacterial or fungal conditions. Anti-parasitic herbs may have to be used in combination with GSE for maximuim effect.

If the condition is chronic, GSE may relieve symptoms but might not totally eliminate the problem. This depends on the nature of the particular organism as well as its location in and beyond the digestive tract. Parasitic infection is not a condition that lends itself to self treatment; consult a physician for the proper course of action.

PERIODONTAL DESEASE (see GUMS)

POISON IVY/POISON OAK

One of the more surprising uses for GSE is in treating contact dermatitis, especially that caused by allergic reactions to poison ivy or poison oak. GSE's effectiveness is based in part upon its extremely astringent nature which helps dry the fluid filled lesions rapidly.

The skin is often broken by persistent scratching and thus becomes susceptible to bacterial infection, especially bacteria of the genus *Staphloccocus*. This type of infection can be extremely serious and may require a pharmaceutical antibiotic. The timely use of GSE can help avoid both the discomfort and potential dangers of contact dermatitis.

Treatment

Mix one ounce GSE with ten ounces of water in a spray bottle and apply to a small area of the affected skin. If a burning sensation results, add ten or more ounces of water; spray liberally over affected areas. Repeat every two hours as needed.

Ringworm

Not a worm, but a fungus of the genus *Trichophytum*, *Microsporum*, or *Epiodermophytum*, this lesion forms a ringlike shape that can appear anywhere on the skin. Ringworm may result from an internal metabolic weakness, poor hygiene or prolonged wearing of wet clothes.

Treatment

Make a solution of GSE as per instructions for poison ivy/poison oak. Spray on affected area several times per day. To increase the effectiveness of the spray, add a tincture of the herb Goldenseal (available at most health food stores). Goldenseal has antifungal properties, but it can temporarily stain the skin so you may wish to add no more than one-half ounce to the solution. It has been reported that a foot powder containing GSE and calcium undecylenate (derived from castor oil) has produced excellent results.

Shaving Itch

These micro-infections are most often caused by a fungus that grows under the skin as a result of small nicks and scratches incurred while shaving. The problem is more likely to occur if razors are reused without having been thoroughly cleansed. Bacterial infections leading to impetigo may also occur.

Treatment

Spray shaved area liberally with a solution of GSE (see CUTS/WOUNDS). When spraying the face, keep eyes closed to prevent irritation. If you intend to reuse the blade, spray it thoroughly with the solution before storing.

SINUSITIS

This condition may stem from a cold, food or inhalant allergies, pressure changes, or even a displacement of the skull bones which could block sinus drainage. If an infection is the cause, a frothy white, yellow, or green discharge may occur; the mucous membranes will be inflamed and extremely tender, therefore extreme care must be taken when using GSE as a sinus douche.

Treatment

Pour one ounce of distilled water into a spray atomizer, add a pinch of salt (solution should have the saltiness of tears), and no more than two drops of GSE. Shake thoroughly and spray gently into the nose, gradually inhaling into the deeper sinuses. Repeat every four hours. If a painful burning sensation occurs, pour out half of the solution and add water to equal one ounce. On the other hand if the original solution is too mild, you may add one or two drops of GSE; shake thoroughly.

Caution: Do not use this treatment for children under twelve without the supervision of a physician.

Sore Thoat

Millions of antibiotic treatments are given every year for throat inflammation. It can be caused by a variety of bacteria, viruses, and even fungi: doctors are most wary when the cause is *B hemolytic strep* . While the bacteria itself poses only a minor threat to the host, it is the allergic reaction to immune complexes created by the body to fight the germ that can cause scarlet fever, rheumatic heart disease, and glomerular nephritis. Serious consequences have been noted in approximately one out of two hundred untreated cases. Because the throat affords easy access, GSE is an ideal adjunct to other treatments; symptomatic relief is often quite rapid with GSE.

Treatment

Thoroughly mix twenty drops of GSE liquid concentrate (or empty two GSE capsules) into six ounces of water (or diluted juice). Gargle deep in the throat for several seconds before spitting out. Repeat until solution is used up. Gargling with GSE can be repeated as often as necessary.

Internal: use the same solution as above and swallow the contents. This insures that areas of the throat inaccessible to gargling are reached and also helps treat the illness systemically.

Caution: If a painful, burning sensation occurs with the recommended solution, reduce the concentration by adding six ounces of water. Consult a physician as soon as possible.

THRUSH

Caused by the fungus Candida albicans, this condition appears as white patches on the oral mucosa of the inner cheeks and lips, tongue, and throat. It most commonly afflicts infants, the elderly, those on antibiotics, and diabetics. Of itself, thrush poses little immediate threat, but it may be a sign that the immune system has been weakened, hence cancer and AIDS patients are prime candidates for thrush. The correct treatment program is determined by the underlying causes of the fungal growth.

Treatment

As with other fungal conditions, GSE can be used topically and internally. As a topical application follow the procedure given for SORE THROAT. Be sure to swish around all areas of the mouth in addition to gargling. If internal treatment is indicated, as it usually is, follow the complete protocol given for Candida (see Ch. 6).

ULCERS (Stomach/Duodenal)

Currently undergoing reevaluation by the medical community, this problem is no longer seen as resulting only from the kind of psychological stress associated with 'Type A' personalities. Veterinarians have long known that ulcers found in pigs caused by the bacteria *Helicobacter pylori* can be cured with the proper antibiotic therapy. This bacteria is also found in the stomachs of twenty to twenty-five percent of humans and is present in more than fifty percent of those who suffer from peptic and duodenal ulcers. This fact recently led scientists to question the entire approach to ulcer therapy. It is now standard procedure to check for the presence of Helicobacter in ulcer cases. When Helicobacter is identified and treated successfully, the sufferer usually finds permanent relief.

Medical treatment for ulcers presently depends largely on two powerful pharmaceutical antibiotics: Ketoconozole and Amoxycillin in combination with the mineral bismuth, a component of Pepto Bismol (Tm). Holistic practitioners, in their attempt to avoid the use of pharmaceutical antibiotics (Ketoconozole is toxic to the liver even in moderate doses), have had some success with various herbal combinations which include bismuth and GSE.

Treatment

Since ulcerated areas are very sensitive to acidic irritation, extreme care must be taken when using GSE. Therefore it is recommended that one begin with the GSE powder. Empty one capsule into twelve ounces of juice or water and drink with one meal per day. Do not swallow the capsule whole; it may cause irritation.) If no irritation occurs after three days use, take with meals twice per day. Continue to increase the dosage every three days by one capsule until a maximum dose of six per day is reached. Decrease dose if burning occurs. A preparation containing bismuth may hasten recovery. Proper attention to diet, especially in regard to food allergies, is also required for maximum benefit.

Caution: Stomach and duodenal ulcers are potentially lethal conditions. Treatment with or without GSE should always be supervised by a physician.

VOMITING (see NAUSEA)

WARTS

Scientists believe that most warts result from the activation of viruses that are either introduced to or lay dormant in the body. The virus uses it own genetic information and our body cells to grow tissue. Obviously its idea of healthy tissue is very different from that of the host. As a result, while a wart is part of the host, it is in fact more like a foreign invader. The aim then, is to treat the offended tissue by removing it.

Since GSE is acidic and antiviral it is not surprising that people have provided positive feedback regarding the use of GSE in the treatment of warts. Warts that grow inward from the skin surface such as plantar warts found on the soles of the feet, have deep roots and can be resistant to topical treatment with GSE though some people have reported sucess. Pedunculated warts, those with a stem or stalk, rise above the surface of the skin and are often more vulnerable to the effects of GSE.

Treatment

Before attempting to treat a wart, consult a licensed physician for a proper diagnosis. Certain skin conditions which may seem like a wart to the untrained eye may in fact be precancerous or cancerous lesions. These should be treated only by a medical expert. Do not use GSE to treat warts located in or around the eyes or genitals; it may cause severe irritation.

Warts are one of the few clinical conditions for which GSE liquid concentrate can be used full strength. Using a cotton swab, carefully apply GSE to the wart making sure to treat all areas, especially the base and stem if possible. Cover with an adhesive bandage to prevent transfer of the GSE to the eyes by the fingers. Repeat two to three times per day; several weeks of treatment may be required for optimal results.

8

ANIMAL HEALTH CARE WITH GRAPEFRUIT SEED EXTRACT

THE AMERICAN HOLISTIC Veterinary Medical Association now boasts over five hundred members as an ever increasing number of veterinarians incorporate holistic health concepts into their practices. Many of these physicians have experienced the same excellent results with GSE as reported in human health care. Consider the words of Stephen Reeve Blake Jr. D.V.M. of San Diego, California,

> *I have found it (GSE) effective in the treatment of Giardia, ear infections, and superficial pyoderma (skin infections). I have also used GSE to purify meat so that I can feed my patients raw meat and not worry about food poisoning....I have used GSE for canker sores,*

> *gum infections and tonsilitis in animals, as a
> vaginal douche for breeding horses (to pre-
> vent infection) and to prevent foot rot in
> horses.*

Philadelphia veterinarian, Dr. Dava Kalsa, has used GSE extensively in her holistic practice. Because ear infections in cats, when caused by fungus, can prove highly resistant to treatment, Dr. Kalsa was particularly interested in GSE's antifungal properties. She says,

> *GSE has proven itself to be extremely depend-
> able and effective while adhering to the crite-
> ria of a natural, non-toxic modality.*

Pat McKay, author of *It's Reigning Cat and Dogs*, has devoted her life to researching the benefits of herbal and homeopathic remedies for animals. Based on en-thusiastic reports from readers, Ms. McKay avidly sup-ports further research into the potential of GSE for animal health care. On the feeding of cats and dogs, Ms. McKay writes,

> *All poultry must be treated with Grapefruit
> Seed Extract to avoid the possibility of Salmo-
> nella, a bacteria that can cause food poison-
> ing. GSE can also be used as a natural preser-
> vative.*

As regards poultry, exciting news was issued in 1984 by the National Veterinary Science Laboratory of Ames, Iowa. Based upon their research,

> *Grapefruit Seed Extract is approved as a disinfectant at a 1:512 dilution for use in the Avian Influenza Eradication Program.*

Further evidence of GSE's relevance in the care of farm animals comes from the USDA Plum Island Animal Disease Center. The Department of Agriculture concluded that viruses causing foot and mouth disease (FMD) and African swine fever (ASF) were deactivated when GSE was used at a dilution of one part per hundred. Swine vesicular disease (SVD) virus was more resistant—it required a concentration of one part in ten for deactivation.

Now that many professionals have found GSE beneficial to cats, dogs, birds, and farm animals, we are hearing reptile and amphibian enthusiasts asking how GSE might be of use to the furless, featherless crowd. It has long been known that pet turtles harbor Salmonella, a bacteria that not only threatens the animal, but humans as well. Since GSE is effective against Salmonella in a laboratory setting, GSE as a treatment for reptiles is an exciting possibility for those concerned with our shell-toting friends.

One of those concerned is Linda Rose Cherney of Los Angelos, a fervent voice in the effort to save the endangered California desert tortoise. Ms. Cherney described to me how these ancient and wonderful animals are threatened by man's encroachment into their habitat and by people collecting them as pets. Her research on the treatment of sick and injured tortoises has revealed yet another arena in which GSE can demonstrate its effectiveness. In Ms. Cherney's opinion,

> *"It appears that Grapefruit Seed Extract can be useful in rehabilitating injured and sick turtles and tortoises. Some people have reported astounding recoveries when natural remedies, especially GSE, are used appropriately. Excellent results have been reported in treating wounds, and cuts; runny nose syndrome, a common but potentially deadly condition, is responding to a combination of GSE and other herbs."*

Back on the Farm

My dog Julie (a ten-year old Cocker Spaniel/Basset Hound mix) has benefited from GSE on many occasions. Like most dogs with drooping ears, Julie is prone to ear infections. By cleaning her ears once a month with a very dilute solution of GSE (two or three drops—

no more—thoroughly mixed into one ounce of water or vegetable glycerine), we have been able to avoid ear infections and their telltale odor.

When Julie and I take our daily hike in the woods she often gets wet. Her reward is a "doggy odor." That odor results more from bacteria and fungi growing on the skin and fur than from the natural odor of a dog. I spray her with a three percent solution of GSE in water making sure to keep it away from her eyes. Within minutes Julie is presentable enough to pay her respects to my patients. But sometimes as a result of digestive upset, her foul breath makes them cringe. It's time to empty two or three GSE capsules into her food. After a few days the improvement is dramatic—she's practically kissable!

Sometimes Julie decides to dine out on an old animal carcass; vomiting and diarrhea may ensue so I give her three capsules of GSE directly down her throat and drinking water (no food). Depending on the severity of symptoms, I may repeat the dosage in two or three hours. She responds remarkably well to this treatment and since I can't trust Julie to learn from her mistakes, I always keep a bottle of GSE capsules nearby.

My parrot Darby spends a good deal of time outdoors during the summer interacting with three ring neck doves, as well as visiting sparrows, chipmunks and squirrels. He enjoys this freedom but it puts him at a greater risk of illness from contact with his friends. For this reason I add one or two drops of GSE to his drinking water each day. I also add 20 drops of GSE to the drinking water of my small flock of five Bantam roosters—it keeps them vigorous. (If the bitterness discourages drinking, use a small amount of powder instead.)

One summer's day I was dismayed to see Darby's right thigh bleeding profusely. Perhaps he got caught by a jagged piece of wire. As I contemplated applying a tiny torniquet, I suddenly remembered a patient of mine who had successfully used GSE in combination with Calendula (marigold) extract to stop the bleeding of a deep wound. I added a few drops of each extract to two ounces of water and gave Darby's leg an herbal shower.

He seemed to take comfort from the treatment but more remarkably his bleeding stopped almost instantaneously. I put him on his perch and when I returned several minutes later there was no sign of bleeding. The next day his thigh was perfectly healed. We were both impressed.

My respect for GSE was heightened further by a report from Florence, a nutritionist who had worked in my office. Florence's cat, Big Guy, had a persistent cough and low grade fever. After several courses of antibiotics and no improvement, Big Guy was found to be suffering from a deadly form of feline leukemia. He had lost his appetite and drank water only sporadically; it seemed he only had a few weeks to live. Florence knew of GSE and decided to give it a try. She gave him two capsules twice daily. Within one week, to everyone's surprise, Big Guy's appetite returned. He put on weight and his cough and fever subsided. He even became affectionate again. GSE did not cure the underlying condition but it did allow Big Guy to live in relative comfort for the last few months of his life.

Although it is imperative to consult a licensed veterinarian before taking it upon oneself to begin a therapeutic program, GSE certainly opens up many options for a holistic approach to animal health care.

9

GRAPEFRUIT SEED EXTRACT IN COMMERCIAL, AGRICULTURAL, AND INDUSTRIAL APPLICATIONS

THE POWER OF GRAPEFRUIT SEED EXTRACT extends far beyond personal health care. We are now seeing a multitude of possibilities for commercial, agricultural, and industrial applications. This brief look at some of these uses is a testament to the creative imagination of scientists, farmers, and business people concerned with the integrity of their products and the well-being of both society and the environment.

COMMERCIAL USES

Since the early 70's there has been a steady increase in the demand for natural cosmetics, soaps, and lotions. The use of herbal extracts in these products has increased the need to control bacterial and fungal growth. Obviously a toxic preservative would destroy the integrity of an otherwise safe product. When researchers at cosmetic manufacturer Este Lauder discovered that only a few drops of GSE in several ounces of skin cream were required to prevent the growth of destructive microoganisms, they no doubt felt their prayers were answered. Naturally, many other companies soon followed suit.

ProGest (Tm) a popular progesterone cream (derived from the wild yam) has successfully employed GSE as a natural preservative. Researchers in the cosmetic industry who know GSE, have invariably praised GSE's ability to control bacteria. Dr. Steven Hernandez, a chemist with Topiderm Inc., N.Y. and a highly respected formulator of skin care products states,

> *while slightly more expensive, GSE is as good, perhaps better than any chemical preservative on the market today.*

Other innovative uses for GSE include:
- An air filter impregnated with GSE liquid concentrate to control airborne mold.
- A spray containing GSE for cleaning cutting boards
- In hot tubs and swimming pools to reduce the need for high levels of chlorine and bromine

AGRICULTURAL USES

At about the same time the cosmetic industry was discovering GSE, farmers and shippers of fruit and vegetables were also learning of its potential. In tropical climates, fungi and bacteria grow rapidly—a fact that threatens the economic viability of some crops. Although chemical sprays or irradiation will retard the growth of microbes, the public is beginning to question the safety of these methods. In test after test, GSE significantly reduced germ growth on fruit and vegetables and thus extended their shelf life. Many consumers report that a dilute spray of GSE (approximately twenty drops per pint of water), extends the shelf life of produce, especially the various types of berries.

In 1989 farmers in the U.S. and Europe began adding GSE liquid and powder to the water and feed of poultry and fish in an attempt to reduce the loss of livestock from infectious diseases. The results were so good that many environmentally conscious farmers have now initiated this practice. These farmers also report another interesting benefit of GSE. It is known that modern farming techniques have significantly increased the prevalence of E. coli and Salmonella in poultry and fish: every year thousands of people suffer food poisoning caused by these bacteria. Farmers are now reporting a significant decrease in E. coli and Salmonella with the use of GSE. It appears that this remarkable antimicrobial is an ecologically sound solution to some of the health problems created by modern farming techniques.

INDUSTRIAL USES

In its role as a disinfectant, GSE is finding many industrial applications, particularly in hospital hygiene. Jerry Skidmore, laundry manager of several hospitals in Florida, states,

> *I have thirty years of experience in the laundry industry and it is only since using GSE that I have the peace of mind and assurance that patients in our hospitals have complete protection from fungal and bacterial infections associated with linen. Furthermore, GSE imparts a fresh and clean smell to the laundry.*

John R. Carson, microbiologist at Armadillo Environmental Services found that GSE could "effectively be used as a disinfectant for domestic wastewater effluent...at an application rate of 2.9 pounds of liquid GSE per million gallons of wastewater." Researchers at Brigham Young University support this finding; regarding the effectiveness of GSE on ten selected fungi and bacteria they concluded that for most of the microorganisms tested "five hundred parts per million of

GSE (approximately one drop in four ounces of water) proved effective within ten minutes."

Two of the most extensive studies on GSE's potential as a disinfectant compared GSE with some of the most popular commercial disinfectants. In November of 1994 the Southern Research Institute completed a study that compared a GSE disinfectant to a leading commercial disinfectant against the following pathogenic germs:

Staphylococcus aureus

Streptococcus pyrogenes

Streptococcus fecalis

Streptococcus pneumonia

Klebsiella pneumonia

Proteus vulgaris

Pseudomonas aeruginosa

Salmonella choleraesuis

Escherichia coli

Candida albicans

Trichophyton mentagrophytes

Herpes simplex virus type 1

Influenza virus type A2

After vigorous study, the Southern Research Institute concluded that GSE proved twice as effective as the commercial formula for inhibiting the above named microorganisms.

Similiar results were obtained when GSE was compared with isopropyl alcohol, perhaps the most frequently used disinfectant in hospitals. But the studies comparing GSE with chlorine bleach and colloidal silver are the most impressive. Bio Research Laboratories of Redmond, Washington, tested GSE, a commercial chlorine bleach, and colloidal silver against Candida albicans, Staphylococcus aureus, Salmonella typhi, Streptococcus faecium, and E. coli. Again, GSE proved itself superior,

> *All microorganisms tested were inhibited with moderate levels of GSE liquid disinfectant. High levels of chlorine bleach inhibited the test organisms, but moderate levels were not effective. Because the GSE liquid was inhibitory at much lower levels, it may be assumed that it is ten to one hundred times more effective than chlorine against the organisms used in this study. On average, GSE proved to be ten times more effective than the colloidal silver.*

These test results are very encouraging, especially considering the environmental dangers posed by the use of chlorine which has the potential to create highly toxic compounds by combining with other chemicals.

The number of non-clinical uses for GSE will surely grow as the public learns of its powerful antimicrobial capabilities.

10

HOUSEHOLD AND OTHER USES FOR GRAPEFRUIT SEED EXTRACT

THE POWERFUL ANTIMICROBIAL properties GSE makes it a versatile cleanser for a broad range of household and outdoor applications. Following are some typical as well as unusual applications for GSE that illustrate its excellent potential.

Note: all suggested uses are based on a fifty/fifty mix of GSE (see explanation following Table 1, Ch. 2).

AIR CONDITIONERS/AIR PURIFIERS

Just as air conditioner ducts harbor germs (a verified cause of deadly Legionaire's disease), so do the filters. Cleaning these filters as well as those of air purifiers on a regular basis with GSE can help reduce the dangers of airborne mold, mildew, and bacteria.

Suggestion: In a spray bottle, mix one teaspoon of GSE with sixteen ounces of water. Spray filter elements once each week; allow to dry before using.

CAMPING

A bottle of GSE liquid concentrate is an invaluable addition to any first aid kit. It can be used to help preserve food (see FOOD RINSE), as a first-aid spray for cuts and wounds (see CUTS/WOUNDS), as a body deodorant, and as an ecologically safe dish washing cleanser. For water decontamination see Ch. 7, PARASITIC INFECTIONS.

CUTTING BOARDS

Nowhere in the home is the risk of food poisoning from microbial contamination as great as it is from the cutting board. Plastic boards, though less porous, may be a greater health threat since wooden ones contain natural, antimicrobial tree resins.

When raw fish or poultry, for instance, is sliced on a cutting board, microbes (e.g., Samonella) can be transferred to the surface. If fruit or vegetables are then sliced on the same surface, severe infection may result.

Suggestion: In a spray bottle, mix one tablespoon of GSE with sixteen ounces of water. Spray onto the surface of the cutting board and let stand for fifteen minutes before rinsing with fresh water.

Food Rinse/Preservation

Although incidents of food poisoning in restaurants have received much media attention in recent years, most illnesses from contaminated beef, fish, chicken, shellfish vegetables and fruit occur in the home. AIDS patients and others with a compromised immune system need to be especially vigilant.

Suggestion: Mix one tablespoon of GSE in one quart of water. Immerse or thoroughly wet food for fifteen minutes; rinse well to remove bitter taste.

Note: The above solution may be added to a spray bottle and used on food to extend shelf life (consumers report excellent results when this procedure is applied to berries of all kinds). Rinse before eating.

Hot Tubs/Swimming Pools

Many people now use GSE to reduce the concentration of chlorine and bromine type chemicals in their hot tubs and swimming pools. Because so many variables exist—temperature, chlorine content, water source, frequency of use, etc—the precise amount of GSE necessary to keep the water free of germs has not yet been determined.

Nevertheless, a ratio of one part GSE to five thousand parts water is generally considered sufficient to control the usual assortment of problematic bacteria. Therefore, a hundred gallon tub would require approximately two and one-half ounces of GSE. This concentration is not likely to irritate the eyes.

Since there are so many variables in this type of application, it is advisable to consult a pool or hot tub expert to better assess your personal requirements.

HUMIDIFIERS

Once the heat in the house goes on for the colder months, it may be necessary to humidify the air to prevent your mouth, lungs, nasal sinuses, and skin from drying out. Unfortunately most cold air humidifiers make excellent breeding grounds for potentially dangerous mold and bacteria which are spread throughout the house by the fine mist from the humidifier.

Suggestion: Empty the humidifier reservoir every day. Add one pint of water and twenty drops of GSE to the tank and cap it. Shake vigorously until a slight foam develops. Let stand five minute before rinsing thoroughly; add fresh water to the tank.

LAUNDRY

A microscopic view of soiled clothing, sheets, and towels reveals a world of microbes we might wish to forget. A typical cold water wash cycle does not guarantee that clothing will be free of these uninvited guests. Chlorine bleach helps but can only be used with colorfast items. Furthermore the use of chlorine bleach may pose an environmental threat.

Suggestion: Add one-half teaspoon GSE to each wash cycle. Clothes will be cleaner and fresher smelling.

MOLD/MILDEW

Wherever dampness accumulates in a house (bathrooms and basements are prime locations) mold and mildew thrive. Old books and antique furniture are also targets. These microbes are not only unsightly and malodorous, but they can produce harmful gases such as formaldehyde, a known carcinogen. Allergies to mold and mildew compromise the health of millions of people each year.

Suggestion: Mix one ounce of GSE in a quart of water. Thoroughly spray or sponge the solution onto the moldy surface or onto those areas that are likely to become contaminated. Repeat often as mold and mildew are notoriously resilient.

Note: If you are concerned about delicate surfaces, apply to an inconspicuous area let stand for ten minutes, then wipe and check for marring.

SHOES/SNEAKERS

Fungi and bacteria feel right at home in your footwear. A solution of GSE as recommended under MOLD/MILDEW should be sprayed lightly into the shoes after each wearing. Wipe dry. As an alternative, distribute the contents of one GSE capsule evenly throughout the shoe. The powder will help dry and decontaminate the shoe.

Toothbrush Cleanser

Your toothbrush removes bacteria and fungi from your mouth but also reintroduces them the next time you brush. Why not get rid of these germs by soaking your toothbrush in a GSE solution?

Suggestion: Soak toothbrush for ten minutes in a solution of five to ten drops of GSE in two ounces of water. Rinse brush with fresh water and allow to dry.

Water Purification

The contamination of water sources by potentially dangerous microbes is a growing problem throughout the world. Many germs are developing a resistance to chlorine; private wells are becoming contaminated at an alarming rate due in part to increased urbanization. As of this writing GSE as a water purifier is still being researched. Therefore GSE should only be used as extra insurance against the possibility of contamination rather than as a first line of defense.

However, reports from travelers suggest that GSE can be used at a ratio of two drops per ounce of water to reduce the risk of drinking water from suspected sources. Flavoring will reduce the bitter taste.

Caution: Certain microbes may be resistant to GSE. Therefore it should not be assumed that GSE will be effective in all cases.

Closing
Words

GRAPEFRUIT SEED EXTRACT has often been referred to as the "Swiss Army knife of germ control." Its versatility is truly extraordinary as attested to by both researchers and consumers who are constantly finding new and innovative uses for both liquid and powder forms. As I have indicated throughout, GSE offers the herbal formulator unparalleled opportunities for creating safe and effective germ control products. But just as GSE offers great opportunities, so does it provide challenges.

Deciphering the precise chemical structure of GSE's active ingredients is of major importance. Understanding its mode of action as well as its limitations is equally compelling. Until more research has been done on safety, the doses of GSE must be kept at moderate levels (since no research has been done regarding pregnancy, "when in doubt, leave it out" holds for expectant mothers). I have often thought that if only 5% of the U.S. health care budget were spent on researching nature's wonderful array of medicines, how much less suffering there would be in the world today. What if medical science was truly open-minded? What if medical research was truly scientific?

The potential of GSE has yet to be realized; it is only one among many such remedies that are challenging the prevailing medical thinking. Fortunately there now exists a critical mass of physicians and consumers who are insisting on safe and effective alternatives to pharmaceutical drugs. To the extent that GSE provides such an alternative, it serves the greater purpose of bringing us back to a deeper appreciation of nature's unlimited potential for health and healing.

The treatments, applications and suggestions presented in this book by no means exhaust GSE's potential—its range of uses is limited only by one's imagination. We welcome innovative ideas and comments from the reader. Send to:

Dr. Allan Sachs
P.O. Box 180
Bearsville, NY 12409

SUGGESTED READING

Buist, Robert. *Food Intolerance.* Garden City Park, N.Y.: Avery Press, 1988.

Connolly, Pat. *The Candida Albicans Yeast-Free Cookbook.* New Canaan, Ct: Keats Publishing 1985.

Crook, William G, *The Yeast Connection/A Medical Breakthrough.* Professional Books.

Garret, Laura. *The Coming Plague.* New York: Farrar, Straus and Giroux, 1994.

Gittleman, Ann Louise. *Guess What Came to Dinner: Parasites and Your Health.* Garden City Park, N.Y.: Avery Press, 1993.

Gittelman, Ann Louise. *Natural Healing For Parasites.* New York: Healing Wisdom Publications, 1995.

Gladwin, Mark. *Clinical Microbiology Made Relatively Simple.* Miami: MedMaster Inc., 1995.

Lipski, Elizabeth. *Digestive Wellness.* New Canaan Ct: Keats Publishing, 1996.

Lorenzi, Shirley. *Candida: A Twentieth Century Disease.* New Canaan Ct: Keats Publishing, 1993.

Randolph, Theron. *An Alternate Approach To Allergies.* New York: Bantam Books, 1980.

Root-Bernstein, Robert. *Rethinking AIDS-The Tragic Cost of a Premature Conclusion.* New York, Free Press, 1993.

Schmidt, Michael. *Beyond Antibiotics.* Berkeley, California: North Atlantic Books, 1995.

Sharamon, Shalila and Baginski, Bodo. *The Healing Power of Grapefruit Seed,* Twin Lakes: Lotus Light Publ., 1996

Staines, Norman et al. *Introducing Immunology.* London: Mosby, 1993.

Trowbridge, John and Walker, Morton. *The Yeast Syndrome.* New York: Bantam Books, 1986.

Articles:

Gittleman, Ann Louise: "The Growing Problem of Parasites", Natural Health, Vol 23, No. 5 page 68, East West Partners, September, 1993.

Newsweek: "The End of Antibiotics", March 28, 1994, page 47-52, New York.

Newsweek: "Outbreak of Fear", May 22, 1995, page 48-55, New York.

New York Times: "From Birth, the Body Houses a Zoo of MIcrobes Working on Its Behalf", October 15, 1996 page C3, New York.

CONVERSION TABLE

All dosages given in this book are based on a fifty/fifty mix of GSE (see explanation following Table 1, Ch. 2). If a concentration other than a fifty/fifty mix (see product label) is used, the dosage must be adjusted as follows:

- Full Strength:[1] twice as potent, therefore use one-half the recommended amount
- 40% Extract: multiply recommended dose by one and one-quarter (e.g.: if 20 drops are recommended then, 20 x 1.25 = 25 drops)
- 33% Extract: multiply recommended dose by one and one-half (e.g.: if 20 drops are recommended then, 20 x 1.5 = 30 drops)

For doses given in teaspoons, tablespoons, or ounces:

1 teaspoon=approx. 130 drops=5ml.

1 tablespoon=3 teaspoons=approx. 390 drops=15+ml.

1 ounce=2 tablespoons=approx. 780 drops=29.5 ml.

1 pint=16 ounces=473 ml.

1 quart=32 ounces=946 ml.

1 gallon=128 ounces=3.78 liters.

---

[1] The 60/40 "Standardized Extract" before further dilution (see explanation following Table 1, Ch. 2).

About the Author

Dr. Allan Sachs, D.C., C.C.N. (Certified Clinical Nutritionist) began his career in health care as a medical researcher at New York's Downstate Medical Center in 1968. Not content with the prevailing medical approach, he undertook the study of chiropractic sciences at New York Chiropractic College and received his Ph.D. in 1978.

Recognized as one of the world's leading authorities on the clinical use of Grapefruit Seed Extract, Dr. Sachs is also the creator of more than twenty-five herbal formulas, currently used by holistic practitioners throughout the world. With his unique combination of chiropractic and nutritional/herbal approaches to healing and his innovative techniques for treating compromised immune sytems, Dr. Sachs has become a pioneer in holistic health. His work has been an inspiration to many natural health practitioners.

Dr. Sachs practices chiropractic and clinical nutrition in upstate New York.

LifeRhythm Publications

John C. Pierrakos M.D CORE ENERGETICS
Developing the Capacity to Love and Heal
With 16 pages of four-color illustrations of human auras corresponding to character structure,
300 pages

John C. Pierrakos, M.D., is a psychiatrist, body-therapist and an authority on consciousness and human energy fields. The focus of his work is to open the "Core" of his patients to a new awareness of how body, emotions, mind , will and spirituality form a unit. Dr. Pierrakos is considered one of the founders of a whole new movement in therapeutic work, integrating body, mind and spirit and this book has become classic.

Bodo Baginski and Shalila Sharamon REIKI
Universal Life Energy
200 pages illustrations

Reiki is described as the energy which forms the basis of all life. With the help of specific methods, anyone can learn to awaken and activate this universal life energy so that healing and harmonizing energy flows through the hands. Reiki is healing energy in the truest sense of the word, leading to greater individual harmony and attunement to the basic forces of the universe. This book features a unique compilation and interpretation, from the author's experience, of over 200 psychosomatic symptoms and diseases

Müller & Günther A COMPLETE BOOK OF REIKI HEALING
Heal Yourself, Others, and the World Around You
192 pages, 85 photographs and illustrations

This book includes the history and practice of Reiki, with photographs and clear instructions for placement of hands in giving Reiki. Brigitte Müller was the first Reiki Master in Europe and she writes about her opening into a new world of healing with the freshness of discovery. Horst Günther experienced Reiki at one of Brigitte's first workshops in Germany, and it changed the course of his life. They share a vision of Reiki and the use of universal life energy to help us all heal ourselves and our world.

Malcolm Brown, Ph.D. THE HEALING TOUCH
An Introduction to Organismic Psychotherapy
320 pages 38 illustrations

A moving and meticulous account of Malcolm Brown's journey from Rogerian-style verbal psychotherapist to gifted body psychotherapist. Dr. Brown developed his own art and science of body psychotherapy with the purpose of re-activating the natural mental/spiritual polarities of the embodied soul and transcendental psyche. Using powerful case histories as examples, Brown describes in theory and practice the development of his work; the techniques to awaken the energy flow and its integration with the main Being centers: Eros, Logos, the Spritual Warrior and the Hara.

Ron Kurtz **BODY-CENTERED PSYCHOTHERAPY:
THE HAKOMI METHOD**
The Integrated Use of Mindfulness, Nonviolence and the Body
212 pages, illustrations
Some of the origins of Hakomi stem from Buddhism and Taoism, especially concepts like
gentleness, compassion, mindfulness, and going with the grain. Other influences come from
general systems theory, which incorporates the idea of respect for the wisdom of each individual as a living organic system that spontaneously organizes matter and energy and se-
lects from the environment what it needs in a way that maintains its goals, programs and
identity. Hakomi is a synthesis of philosophies, techniques and approaches that has its own
unique artistry, form and organic process.

Helmut G. Sieczka **CHAKRA BREATHING**
A Pathway to Energy and Harmony
100 pages Illustrations   Supplemental Cassette Tape Available
A guide to self-healing, this book is meant to help activate and harmonize the energy centers of the subtle body. Through the practice of chakra breathing we can learn to explore
and recognize our innate possibilities, uncovering hidden energy potentials. The breath is
the bridge between body and soul. In today's world as our lives are determined by stressful
careers and peak performance, the silent and meditative moments have become more vital.
We can try to remember our true selves more often, so that our natural energy balances
can be restored. Chakra-breathing enhances this kind of awareness and transformational
work, especially on the emotional and energetic level.

R. Stamboliev **THE ENERGETICS OF VOICE DIALOGUE**
Exploring the Energetics of Transformational Psychology
100 pages
Voice Dialogue is a therapeutic technique based on the transformational model of consciousness. This book approaches the human psyche as a synthesis of experience-patterns which
may be modified only when the original pattern of an experience has been touched, understood and felt from an adult, integrated perspective, developing an "Aware Ego". This book
explores the energetic aspects of the relationship between client and therapist, offering exercises for developing energetic skills and giving case histories to illustrate these skills. This
book is a unique expression of the work of Hal and Sidra Stone Ph.Ds, creators of Voice
Dialogue. Voice Dialogue is taught in the USA and now in many parts of the world.

Fran Brown **LIVING REIKI: TAKATA'S TEACHINGS**
Stories from the Life of Hawayo Takata
110 pages
In this loving memoir to her teacher, Fran Brown has gathered the colorful stories told by
Hawayo Takata during her thirty-five years s the only Reiki Master Teaching. The stories
create an inspirational panorama of Takata's teachings, filled with the practical and spiri-
tual aspects of a life given to healing.

Reinhard Flatischler THE FORGOTTEN POWER OF RHYTHM
TA KE TI NA
160 pages, illustrations   Supplemental CD or Cassette
Rhythm is the central power of our lives; it connects us all. There is a powerful source of rhythmic knowledge in every human being, and as we find our way back to this ancient wisdom, we unite with the essence of our life. Reinhard Flatischler presents his brilliant approach to rhythm is this book, for both the layman and the professional musician.
TA KE TI NA offers an experience of the interaction of pulse, breath, voice, walking and clapping which awakens our inherent rhythm in the most direct way—through the body.

John C. Pierrakos M.D. EROS, LOVE & SEXUALITY
The Unifying Forces of Life & Relationship
130 pages
"The unobstructed flow of the three great forces of life—sexuality, eros, and love—creates our most important source of pleasure. These three forces are simply different aspects of the life force, but when they flow freely they are experienced as one. They generate all activity, all creativity. We feel this force when we are moved by a symphony, a beautiful sunset, or love for another (from the text.) John Pierrakos, the great body-psychotherapist, was a student and colleague of Wilhelm Reich and co-founder of Bioenergetics; he later developed his own therapeutic work, Core Energetics. He lectures and teaches worldwide.

LIFERHYTHM

Connects you with your Core and entire being—guided by
Science, Intuition and Love.
We provide tools for growth, therapy, holistic health and higher education
through publications, seminars and workshops.
If you are interested in forthcoming projects and want to be on our mailing
list, send your address to:

P.O. Box 806   Mendocino CA   95460   USATel: (707) 937-1825
Fax: (707) 937-3052   E-mail: lisycee@mcn.org